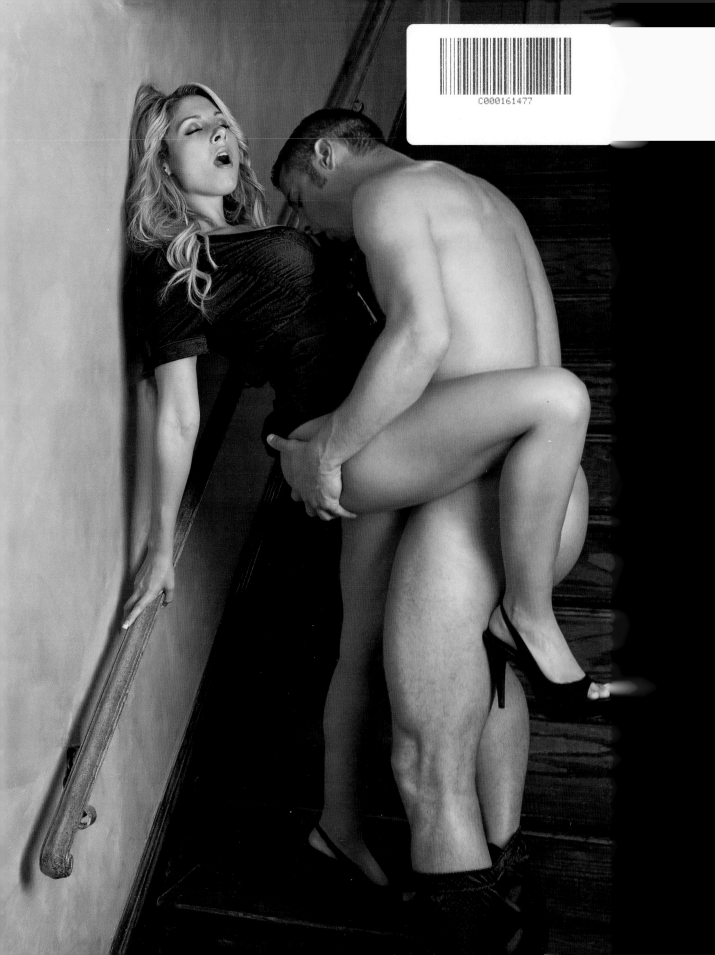

© 2011 Quiver
Text © 2011 Robin Westen
Photography © 2011 Quiver

First published in the USA in 2011 by
Quiver, a member of
Quayside Publishing Group
100 Cummings Center
Suite 406-L
Beverly, MA 01915-6101
www.quiverbooks.com

The publisher maintains the records relating to images in this book required by 18 USC 2257. Records are located at Rockport Publishers, Inc., 100 Cummings Center, Suite 406-L, Beverly, MA 01915-6101.

15 14 13 12 11   1 2 3 4 5

ISBN: 978-1-59233-493-3

Digital edition published in 2011
eISBN-13: 978-1-61058-183-7

Library of Congress Cataloging-in-Publication Data available

Book design by Traffic Design Consultants
Book layout by www.meganjonesdesign.com
Photography by Holly Randall

Printed and bound in Singapore

THE 12 MINUTE SEX SOLUTION

HAVE ELECTRIFYING SEX IN NEW WAYS WITH 75 QUICK AND DIRTY SCENARIOS YOU CAN DO IN 12 MINUTES OR LESS

ROBIN WESTEN

QUIVER

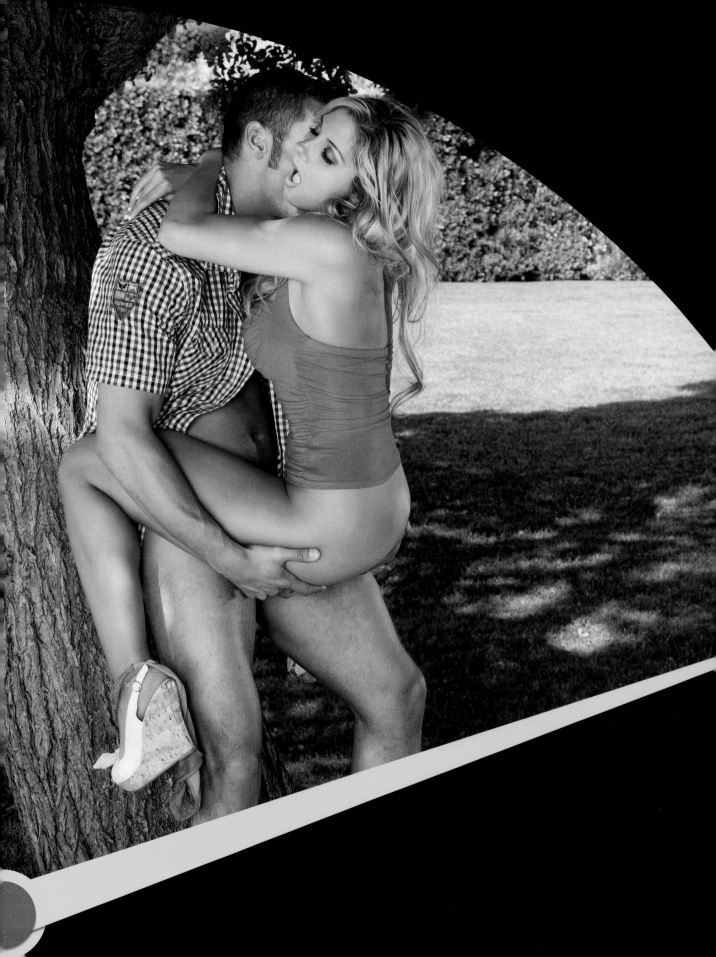

CONTENTS

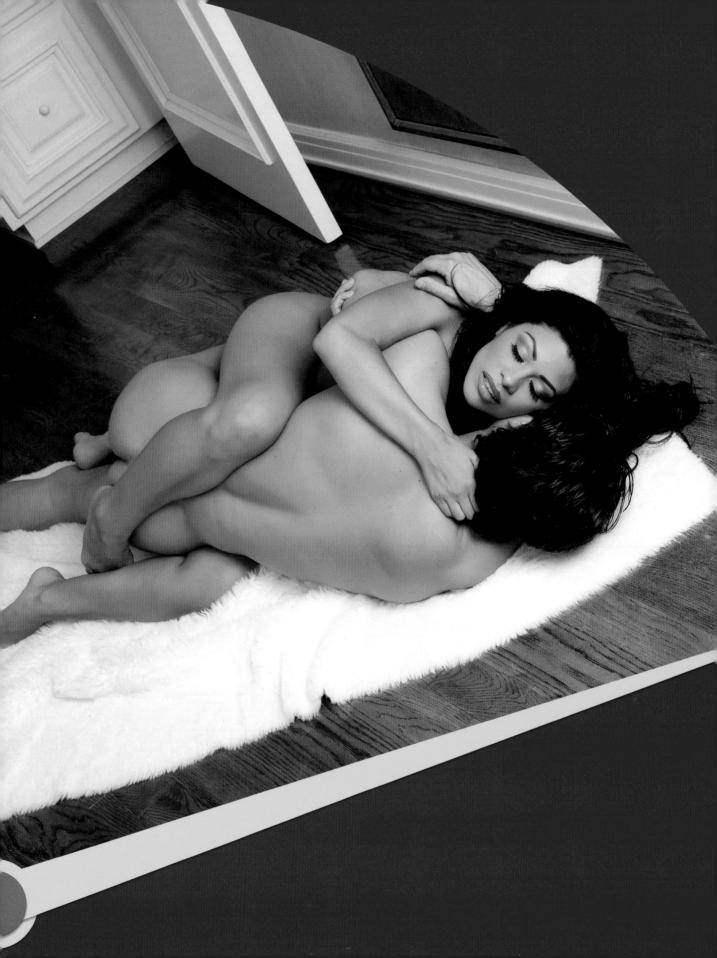

INTRODUCTION

Nearly every time I get together with friends for girl talk, one of them complains about her boring or slim-to-nonexistent sex life. Listen to my flame-haired friend Valerie, for example: "I love my husband like crazy," she tells me in a hush. "But try juggling the needs of a toddler, a job, housework, cooking, and shopping, plus both sets of relatives. Believe me." She sighs. "There's just never enough time or energy left in the day to make love. And if we do, it's just the same-old, same old, in-and-out ho hum."

I nod in agreement but secretly refuse to accept this sad situation. As a sex advice columnist, health writer, and loving wife, I know that at every chance our bodies get to merge with our partner's we're reaffirming our love; there's nothing better. I also know making love whatever way we can, and whenever we can, is always better than turning away from desire. But I'm also a realist. Rather than let myself fantasize about scheduling impossibly long romantic weekends or hard-to-keep weekly date nights, I get to thinking about whether there's a way to have amazing sex even while we're in the midst of checking off our mile-long to-do list.

That's how *The 12-Minute Sex Solution* took seed. A recent scientific study proved both men and women get highly aroused in just 12 minutes or less, so I knew my idea wasn't far-fetched. But studies can take you only so far; I wanted to come up with *real* situations and a PLAY BY PLAY plan that would guarantee stressed-to-the-max couples not only more sex, but better, unforgettable, imaginative, drenching-to-the max sex.

Thanks to an abundance of research, interviews with couples offering practical suggestions and a willingness to try different methods, as well as discussions with experts, I've created 75 scenarios for mind-blowing sexual pleasure, geared specifically to partners who think there's just not enough time in the day for great sex.

The 12-Minute Sex Solution is easy to read and simple to put into action. Chapter 1 is a hands-on manual that instructs couples on the importance of setting the foundation for quick and satisfying sex. In this chapter, couples are encouraged to prepare themselves to once again make sex a priority in their on-the-go lives. After all, great sex doesn't just happen. The 12 tips in chapter 1 are based on research, and they help boost the libido, eroticize the individual, and create an atmosphere and foundation of intimacy and longing for ultra-busy couples.

This chapter also explains the research that is the backbone of *The 12-Minute Sex Solution*. Readers who are juggling busy schedules but want to inject intensity back into their sex lives will understand how and why the activities work and will be encouraged to indulge in these fast and satisfying steps.

Chapters 2 through 5 make up the heart of *The 12-Minute Sex Solution*. They describe the 75 best times to grab nookie while you're taking care of business in the naughtiest locations, sexiest positions, and most erotic pleasure points—along with step-by-step instructions leading to hot-button excitement and urgent climaxes. All the steps are streamlined for pleasure so busy couples can carve out the time they need.

There's no right time or place to make love, but there are plenty of heart-pounding, testosterone-pumping opportunities for couples who want to inject romantic intensity into their hectic lives. Put passion back on your priority list. Read on.

01

HOW TO RECLAIM YOUR SEX LIFE IN 12 MINUTES

YOU'RE NOT ALONE

The number one complaint loving couples express is the frustration that there is *never enough time for sex*. During 2009, sex therapists reported seeing an increase in the number of couples who again and again complained of being too busy, tired, or stressed out to make love. And a recent study from the National Sleep Foundation confirms that among married people or couples living together, one in four adults skips or avoids sex because he or she is too tired to expend the time and energy it takes to do it. This is especially unfortunate because sex releases oxytocin, a stress-relieving/energy-boosting hormone—something we could all use during these hectic days.

There's plenty of evidence showing sex also boosts our physical and mental well-being in other ways. For instance, making love can help burn calories, keep bones healthy, lower cholesterol levels, relieve PMS symptoms, improve circulation, relieve pain and depression, and strengthen the immune system. In fact, a study by Wilkes University showed the more sex couples had, the less often they suffered colds and flus. Most important, exciting sex not only feels fantastic, but it also strengthens and deepens our relationships by creating a bond of intimacy.

So how do you do it? Unless you're the love-struck heroine in a romance novel and your partner is the bare-chested, eight-pack-rippling Fabio, I can tell you this … you *won't* need any of the following: flickering candlelight, scattered rose pedals, silk sheets, champagne poured into crystal flutes, a platter of oysters, an exotic island retreat, a bearskin rug, a roaring fire, a scented bubble bath, Marvin Gaye crooning "Sexual Healing," or twenty-four nonstop hours in the sack. In fact, many sex therapists agree that by the time you stage those kinds of contrived scenarios, the pressure to perform kills the passion.

So what *will* you need?

THE FOUR STEPS

According to my carefully researched plan, you need to take only *four essential steps* to get and give amazing sex in practically no time at all:

Step #1: Nurture arousal
Step #2: Devote 12 minutes (or less) to super-connected sex
Step #3: Turn ordinary activities into gutsy and erotic adventures
Step #4: Hit hot-button positioning for maximum outcome

Step #1: Nurture Arousal

Sex therapists say it's helpful to keep your libido on alert so you can be receptive to sex at a moment's notice. Arousal is a state of sexual excitement that sends messages to our brain, which then creates physical changes and sensations throughout our whole body, particularly our genitals, readying us for sex of any kind. When you're in a state of arousal, follow-through orgasm methods are quicker and easier to achieve.

You don't have to schedule a special time in your busy life to accomplish this. Just follow these suggestions to help you stay aroused even while you dash through your hectic day:

- **Cultivate sexual fantasies during ordinary daily activities**—for example, while you're driving to work or shopping in the supermarket. Sex therapists say visualizing intimacy before engaging in sex heightens your level of arousal. And research has shown that imagining yourself in a sexy situation can stimulate some of the same body sensations as actually being in that situation.

- **Wear sexy underwear (or no underwear)** even when you're not planning on making love.

- **Enjoy erotic literature.** Experts suggest saving pornography for when you're with your partner.

- **Feast on spicy foods,** because hot pepper releases some of the same endorphins as sex does.

- **Add red to your wardrobe or environment.** Chromologists say red is the color of arousal and gets the heart pumping.

- **Soap yourself in the shower the way your lover would.**

- **Cross and uncross your legs while sitting.** Physiologists explain that rubbing your thighs together increases blood flow to your genitals, which gives a tingly, aroused feeling.

- **Masturbate in the bathroom or shower,** or before going to sleep or getting out of bed in the morning. Knowing that you can control your own sexual pleasure with masturbation is something that can transform anyone's experience of sex into something that is *always* positive and pleasurable and *never* limited. Research shows a positive attitude toward masturbation increases rates of arousal.

- **Keep things wet and carry travel-size bottles of lubricant.** Wetter makes for better action—and easier efforts, too. A new study by sexual health researchers at Indiana University found that women who used lubricant in and out of the bedroom reported significantly higher levels of satisfaction and pleasure.

- **Get your heart racing.** You don't have to take up sky diving but do take *some* risks during the day, whether it's volunteering to make a toast at a party or taking a different route home from work. Giving yourself an adrenaline rush spikes the brain's natural amphetamines—dopamine and norepinephrine—thereby making you more aroused.

- **Exercise when you can.** Besides helping you feel good about your body, exercising elevates your mood, increases your stamina, and boosts your libido. Women: Try Kegel exercises to strengthen your pelvic muscles and intensify sexual sensations. You can do these while you're sitting at your desk, waiting on line at the cashier, or washing the dishes.

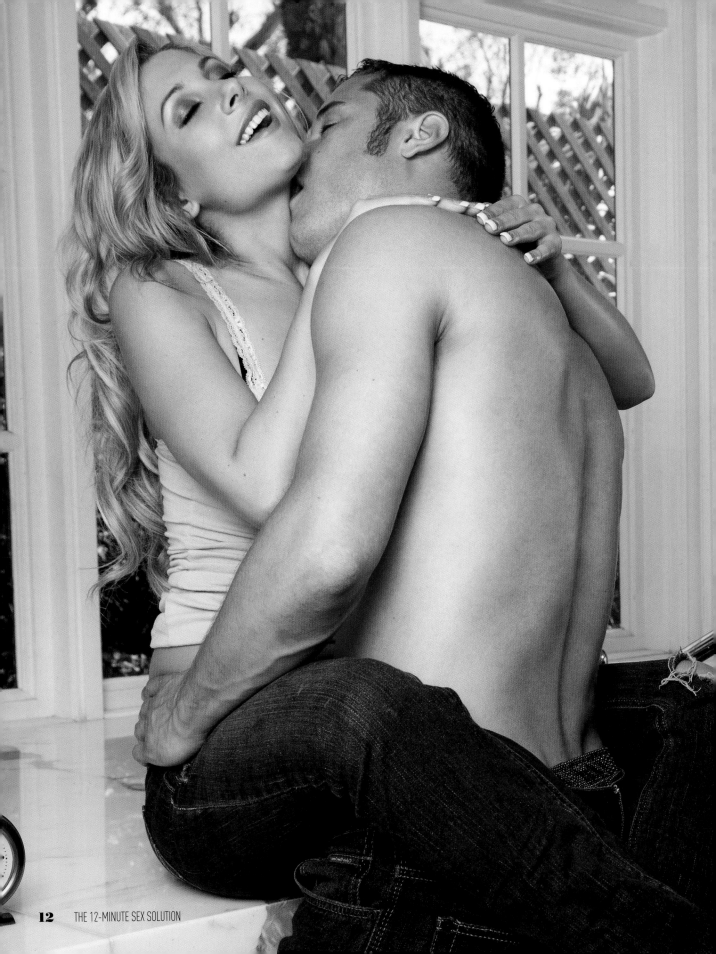

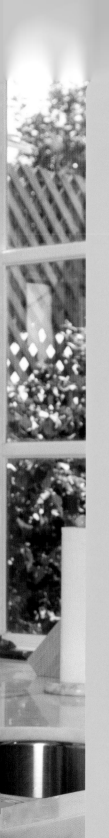

Step #2: Devote 12 Minutes (or Less) to Super-Connected Sex

Do you think 12 minutes just isn't enough time to have delicious, delirious, super-satisfying sex? Well, think again. Recent research at McGill University Health Centre in Montreal, Canada, used thermal imaging to measure increased blood flow to men and women's genital regions. The study concluded that both men and women reach peak arousal in 12 minutes or less; men reach peak sexual arousal in 665 seconds—about 10 minutes—while women arrive at maximal arousal in 743 seconds. The McGill research gives heat to the power of super-charged, fast sex.

And that's the way we like it. According to a survey led by U.S. and Canadian sex therapists, most people believe that 7 to 13 minutes is the "desirable" amount of time to have sex; 3 to 7 minutes is "adequate," and anywhere between 20 to 30 minutes is just "too long." Turns out, couples who are juggling family, careers, and a love life aren't the only ones to appreciate furious, frantic, high-speed sex.

But even 12 minutes can seem like an unattainable eternity when schedules are at a fever pitch, so we suggest couples make a four-pronged pact with their partner that states:

- At least twice a week, I agree to devote 12 minutes out of my day for quick, quality sex.

- I will remain open to making the most out of sexual opportunities that present themselves, no matter what activity I'm engaged in.

- If I'm not in the mood or it's absolutely the wrong time, I will let my partner know.

- I will not take rejection personally but will look forward to the next chance we get.

Step #3: Turn Ordinary Activities into Erotic Adventures

Coming up with ways to fire up lust within 12 minutes while you're working around a tight schedule may seem impossible. Don't bother wrapping your head around it. The *Solution* finds those opportunities for you in the midst of your ordinary day, especially during common activities, which provide *ideal* circumstances for fulfilling your sense of sexual urgency. Among the possibilities: Deliver an amazing blow job in under 10 minutes while your guy is shaving. Make Scrabble sexy. Pull off an unforgettable hand job during halftime. Have sex on the spin-cycle (literally). And dozens more!

To keep desire fired up, we recommend couples engage in at least two erotic activities a week. If it's possible to increase the frequency, don't hold back—be brave and go for it. Research shows the more you get it on, the more you want to get it on, because sex makes testosterone surge through our bodies. (Women have testosterone, too!) And testosterone is the hormone that makes you crave sex.

We also recommend paging through the book together, gazing at the graphic photographs, allowing your imaginations to flow and your libidos to feel the heat. Plan to go over at least two activities a week "in depth," perhaps reading them aloud and then mulling over the PLAY BY PLAYs.

Hopefully you'll know when the time is right to try an activity out. For example, it's probably not the best idea to launch into a sexy striptease while he's in the middle of doing the taxes, or to pounce on her when she's just walked in after a bad day at the office. Communication and awareness of each other's needs are basic keys to an exciting fast encounter.

Step #4: Hit Hot-Button Positioning for Maximum Outcome

Couples should beware not to place too much importance on the orgasm itself; the goal of sex is not necessarily to reach one. Turning the heat up by cuddling for 12 minutes can be just as emotionally satisfying as climaxing. As long as both partners are enjoying themselves and experiencing an intimate connection, there really is no reason to feel pressure to achieve orgasm.

That said, it's *always* fun to have one. It's why the *Solution* gives a PLAY BY PLAY, describing the exact moves to make, positions to take, clothes to wear, and accoutrements needed to turn your partner's heat all the way up to scorching. When you read the PLAY BY PLAYs, visualize the act rather than trying to put them to rote memory. Putting your fantasy into action not only increases arousal, but it also keeps performance anxiety out of the picture.

Remember: *There's no wrong way* to make love. However, the PLAY BY PLAYs explain how to make ordinary daily activities tantalizing, such as feeling the vibration of the dryer on your bare butt, waiting for cupcakes to cool while being playfully smacked with a batter-smeared spoon, allowing your nails to dry as you're bound to the bedpost, or giving a blow job while eating an ice cream cone.

The *Solution* also offers practical tips on penetration, cunnilingus, blow jobs, hand jobs, role-playing, dirty talk, masturbation, pleasure points, pornography, sexting, stripteases, bondage, spanking, and much, much more. As in any sexual activity, be adventurous—but go only as far as you both feel comfortable.

Note: Be daring, but if you don't want to get caught in the act, or caught directly after it, keep these suggestions in mind:

- Watch the clock. In the heat of the moment, it's tempting to extend your quickie into a *longie*, but be aware of how much time you have and how much time you'll need to freshen up.

- Make sure your spot is secret. A locked room is ideal, but if that's not an option, then you'll want to find a place that's out of sight and earshot, where no one is likely to barge in. The *Solution* offers plenty of ideas, including a secluded closet or bathroom, the top-floor stairwell of a building, or the back of a parked car.

- Zip and button up. Make sure you and your co-conspirator double-check your clothes to make sure all zippers and buttons are fastened properly. Nothing says "we just had sex" like misaligned buttons.

- Have a good excuse if you're late. Make it seem like you really hurried— to explain the flush in your cheeks.

- Don't kiss and tell. Secrecy keeps it hot.

Now that you've been primed to get the most out of *The 12-Minute Sex Solution*, browse through the rest of the book and let your imaginations soar. If you need it, want it, or are simply thinking about it, you'll find the time, location, and best PLAY BY PLAYs to make sex better—and bolder—than ever before.

02

AT-HOME ENTERTAINMENT
Staying in for Sexual Satisfaction

The key to a happy and fulfilled sex life is the ability to nurture a spirit of adventure and fun. But does that mean you need to take a trip down the Amazon River or hang glide over the Alps to experience the freedom and connection of daring lovemaking? *No way.* The most intimate, spontaneous relations can be experienced right in your own home, where you are, on the spot, and with little or no preparation. It's all about making the most of available opportunities to express your sexuality and desire.

In this chapter, you'll learn how to turn homebound activities like watching television, showering, eating dinner, taking a nap, and reading the newspaper into memorable, audacious, erotic escapades. You'll get to enjoy fast, furious fun in every room in your house, from the bathroom and backyard to the kitchen, living room, and, okay, the bedroom, too. And, you'll get the PLAY BY PLAYs for amazing orgasms atop a variety of furniture, from the sofa, desk chair, and workbench to the bathtub and the kitchen counter. All of this gives new meaning to the term *homebodies*.

FYI: Ladies, when you're home, keep your socks on during sex. According to the results of a study in the Netherlands, women who wear socks orgasm 80 percent of the time compared with barefoot women, who orgasm 50 percent of the time.

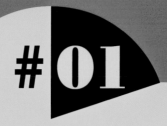

HALFTIME DEEP-THROAT PASS

Oh, football. If you're a woman, you probably feel invisible. Well, you'll get him cheering for *you* with this powerful play: a deep-throat blow job. Grab hold of him *now* and make the most of the break. FYI: Football half-times last 15 minutes. How perfect is *that*?

Estimated time: 12 minutes (leaving time to refill the snack bowl)
What you'll need: a recliner or couch, a can-do spirit

THE PLAY BY PLAY

1. Before you do *anything*, assure your sports fan that he'll be back to the game before his team returns to the field. This isn't a game where overtime is allowed.

2. Be bold and force him to lie back and enjoy halftime while you unzip his pants and pull out his cock and balls. (This should put any of his hesitation to rest.)

3. Deep-throating is an erotic act in which you put your man's entire erect penis deep into your mouth in such a way as it slides down your throat. It was popularized by the 1972 porn film *Deep Throat*, but in many cases it's easier said than done.

4. Not surprisingly, men love deep-throating, but lots of women find it difficult to perform because to do it you have to suppress the natural gag reflex. Your gag reflex is a soft palate in the back of your throat. Though its designed to stop you from choking, your gag reflex's power can be overcome by your desire to deep-throat. Good news: One-third of the population doesn't even have a gag reflex! For them (and maybe you), deep-throating will be no problem.

A few other suggestions:

- Having him on his back allows you to better control his movement by using your forearms to push him down if he begins to thrust to a point that is uncomfortable and you start to, uh, gag.

- You can also gently tug on his testicles to let him know he needs to slow it down. Don't do this too hard, though, because the last thing you want to do is cause any discomfort. Offer just enough pressure to signal to pull back. He'll know what you're trying to do.

- If, despite your best efforts, your gag reflex is still triggered, or if he is well endowed (lucky you!) and deep-throating is a challenge, fake it. Here's how: With your hand, make a fist around the shaft of your lover's penis and rest your little finger on his pubic bone. Move your mouth and up and down the head and upper shaft of his penis while moving up and down with your hand at the same time. This offers a similar sensation to deep-throating without the angst of gagging.

5. Now back to the game!

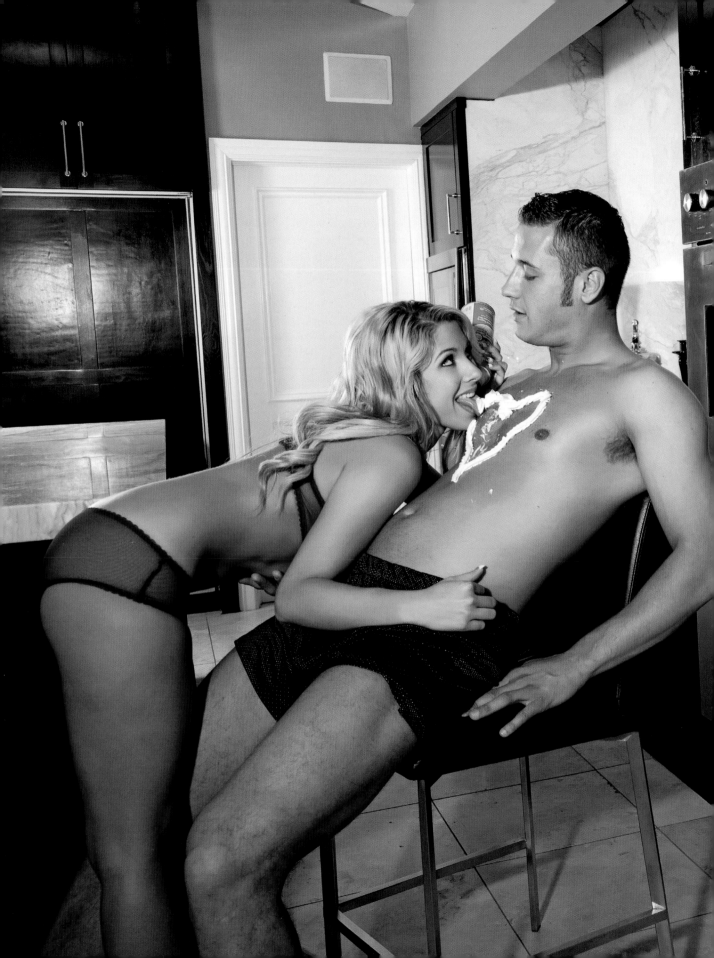

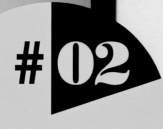

JUST DESSERTS BLOW JOB

Since the kids are fast asleep and you're taking the time to enjoy dessert anyway, why not make it doubly delectable? The link between food and sex is powerful. Yummy food (especially if it's chocolate) triggers the pleasure centers of the brain, releasing the bliss-creating chemical dopamine. Getting lewd with food and offering a tasty blow job is bound to reap sweet appreciation. Go ahead: Play with your food.

Estimated time: 10 minutes or less
What you'll need: three of your favorite sweet ingredients that can be smeared safely on your man's penis (think chocolate syrup, whipped cream, caramel sauce—all at room temperature), a hearty appetite

THE PLAY BY PLAY

1. Let's hope your honey has a sweet tooth. If he does, place a delectable dessert in front of him and let his eyes feast on it. Just tease him, though. Before he has a chance to dig in, move the plate and sit on his lap. Squirming is always a good idea, because any movement helps arousal. There's a reason why men dig those lap dances.

2. Once he's hungering for more, lean over and put the plate on the floor. Then slide off his lap and get on your knees.

3. Without any discussion, unzip his pants and tug his underwear and pants to his ankles.

4. Put his penis in your mouth and hold it there. Resist moving your tongue or sucking. Remember: This is about sweet temptation and teasing. There's more to come.

5. When you feel him hardening, with one hand, reach for the dessert plate. Keep your other hand around the base of his shaft so you don't lose momentum.

6. Slowly release your mouth and smear the dessert concoction on his penis from the tip of the head, all along his shaft, to the base.

7. Finally, it's time for your just desserts. Enjoy your sweet with gusto, licking his penis, allowing your tongue to make circles around this head as if you were enjoying a chocolate-covered banana— no bites, just licks. Moan with delight, and go for more ... don't count calories. Remember: You'll burn most off with your passion.

8. When you feel he's about to burst, stop smearing and slide his entire penis in your mouth. Suck rhythmically until he reaches climax.

9. To add an unforgettable topping, hold his penis in your mouth for a few more seconds. After you let it slide out, lick it again. Then scoop more dessert and put it in your mouth and lean into him, offering a last soulful tongue kiss.

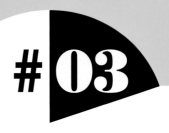

#03

TUB-COOLING FROLIC

Oops! The bathwater is too hot. While you're waiting for it to cool off, take a different sort of dip. The bathroom is already warm and steamy. Ask your partner to join you, then lock the door and get naked.

Estimated time: 7 minutes
What you'll need: a towel or bath mat to spread on the floor, lube, a moderate level of flexibility

THE PLAY BY PLAY

1. This is a good time for ladies to get down and dirty take the lead. Place the bath mat on the floor, perpendicular to the tub with the narrower side touching the edge of it.

2. Lie on top of the mat with your legs apart, straight and extended upward like a pair of scissors. Your butt should be facing the wall of the tub, as the tub rim will offer you support. Although this might sound like you need to be Gumby to get into this position, it's really not difficult to manage. The tub will give you lots of support and the steam will keep you flexible.

3. Men, now share the mat with your lover, sitting between her thighs with your back against the wall of the tub.

4. Either one of you can generously apply lubrication to his penis and your vagina. This is really important because even though steamy air feels wet, the heat in the air can dry out genitals.

5. Now you're both in a perfect position for the next step, and your guy can gently penetrate you using his forearms to support you both.

6. Here's a hint for women: If you want to tighten your grip, then flex your toes. It will make it feel as if you're holding him tightly inside of you.

7. Remain still while he enters you shallowly to begin with—and then more deeply. Guys: Alternate your pace but keep it gentle. Remember that the tub is a hard surface with no give.

8. Another suggestion for women who want to maximize their intensity: Squeeze your thigh and pelvic muscles together as he thrusts. This will help build your orgasm.

9. Hey, guys, don't feel left out. Contract your PC (pubococcygeal) muscles too, to give you an extra dose of pleasure.

10. After you've both enjoyed coming, slide into your now perfectly comfortable and soothing bathwater. Room for two?

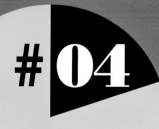

SWING TIME

It's a stunning spring day, and you're luxuriating in the hammock. *What?! You're alone??* Don't waste this chance! Call your partner over. A hammock can be a great accessory for sex, giving you and your mate an almost weight-less feeling. Indeed, there are a number of companies that sell "love swings" for this very purpose, but you can use the one you're on for a risky encounter.

Estimated time: 10 minutes
What you'll need: a hammock, lube, trust, a fairly good sense of balance, a secluded area, bug spray if the mosquitoes are hungrier than you are

THE PLAY BY PLAY

1. Start off with some stability—otherwise, hammock sex can feel too out of balance to be pleasurable. It's better if your gal takes the bottom position and lies down perpendicularly in the middle of the swing; in other positions, you both risk tumbling out.

2. Now that you're settled in, lift up her skirt or pull down her pants and panties and liberally apply lube to her vagina. The heat of the sun on her pussy will make this sensation especially soothing.

3. Since you're in the great outdoors, hopefully your hammock is hung in a remote area away from prying eyes. The perfect technique for hammock sex is the *Lataveshta*, which is a position in the *Kama Sutra* involving a tangling of limbs done with guys on top. It's an ideal position for intimacy because it features slow, sensual movements. It's also known as the Clinging Creeper (think vines around a pole).

4. Guys, even though the idea of great outdoor sex is irresistible, ease into it slowly. Hammock sex requires a bit more caution.

5. Slip your penis into your lover's vagina. If you're not yet hard, stroke your cock until it gets harder, and then guide it inside—though guys can usually get it up easily in the great outdoors, especially if they're into the fantasy of getting caught doing the dirty.

6. You can spend time having "simple" missionary sex in this position, or ...

7. ... Move straight into the *Lataveshta* position by entwining your arms and legs. Women, it's your move next: From the missionary position, wrap your legs around his and hook your ankles, locking him in. Then twist your arms around his arms.

8. Practice a slow, gentle rocking movement. This position restricts movement to shallow thrusts because your limbs lock your bodies tightly together. It's totally ideal for hammock sex because there are no jarring movements.

9. Synchronize your breathing with the sways of the hammock to heighten your intimate connection. Breathing together will help your bodies heave and peak at the same time.

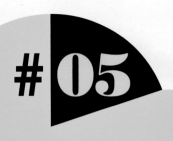

#05

THE BIG *OM*

Millions of people around the world find the time in their busy schedules to practice yoga. A majority of them practice not only at private studios but also in their homes. As you know, one of the fundamental poses is Downward-Facing Dog. Need we say more?

Estimated time: 3–5 minutes
What you'll need: a yoga mat, some familiarity with simple yoga poses, lube

THE PLAY BY PLAY

1. Yogis, skip the organic cotton outfit and do this pose in your birthday suit. Pretend you need his advice and ask your man to check out your Downward-Facing Dog position. Seeing you nude, he'll get the drift that you want more from him than a posture correction.

2. This pose involves placing your hands and feet shoulder- and hip-width apart on the floor with your butt in the air, creating a sort of triangular/bridge shape with your body. Your back should be straight or very slightly arched and you should feel firmly rooted to the floor.

3. For an even more sex-accessible pose, spread your legs slightly wider than hip-width and, if possible, arch your back a little more. This will allow your partner to penetrate and access your G-spot more easily. Due to your somewhat upside-down position, this pose allows blood to flow to different parts of your body, especially your head. It also offers a completely new visual vantage point.

4. Ask your lover to help you out here. Tell him that the only way you'll know if you're in perfect alignment is if his cock can reach your G-spot. Hand over the lube you've got by the side of your mat.

5. Wait for him to get aroused while he spreads the lube on your vagina. That should be after about five deep breaths.

6. Once he's inside you, try shifting your weight from one leg to the other to see whether it allows for deeper penetration or more direct stimulation.

7. Because this position requires that both you and your partner have good balance, you may want to modify it by dropping to your knees, bringing you closer to the more traditional doggie-style position but still maintaining an arched back and spread legs.

8. Say "O ... O ... *Ommmmm!*"

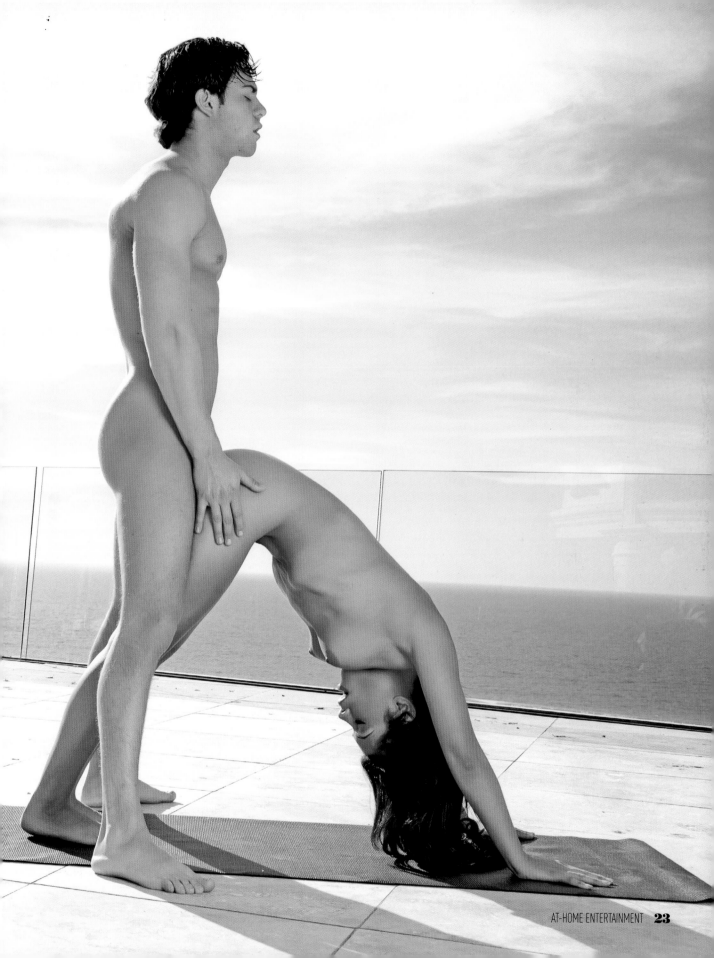

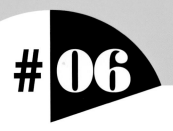

DIRTY, DANGEROUS SCRABBLE

Scrabble has been around for seventy-two years. But if you're a couple of Scrabble fiends, there's no reason to stick to the same old rules. This new twist will get your sexual juices flowing—and fast.

Estimated time: 12 minutes
What you'll need: Scrabble game, an erotic mind-set, agreed-upon new rules, a dirty-word vocabulary

THE PLAY BY PLAY

1. Once you get started, you'll probably find that it's not only easy but also lots of fun to create your own sexy games. Any board game can be a turn-on for you and your partner. Just make a few steamy modifications to the current rules, and *voilà*! But be sure to agree on the new rules before you begin. For example, when it comes to Dirty, Dangerous Scrabble, you may need to allow words that are more than seven letters or can't be found in a standard dictionary. You can also change the way it's played, the rewards for winning, the penalties for losing, or whatever else you wish. Changing the rules will go a long way toward creating your very own sexy game.

2. For Dirty, Dangerous Scrabble, agree to use only erotic words. Expand your vocabulary to include not only parts of the body or the usual sexy verbs but also words like *bite*, *slap*, *scratch*, *bondage*, etc., just to steam things up.

3. After you've been aroused by the dirty language and innuendo, you can decide whether you want to keep on playing or instead fall to the floor and step up the intensity by putting your words into action.

4. If you're both game, use some of the sexy words you've placed on your Scrabble board. Dirty talking can be a big turn-on.

5. You might want to keep up your competitive spirit by teasing each other with light scratching, biting, and pinching. When you use just the right pressure, you can add a threat of danger without inflicting pain. Start lightly and intensify pressure gradually. Gentle biting or pinching of nipples on both sexes usually gets juices flowing.

6. If you feel yourself on the verge of coming and think your partner may be lagging behind, increase the intensity but always play it safe. Don't get too carried away. If one of you says "Enough" or "Stop," well, you'll have to cease *immediately*.

7. Another adaptation of sexy word games is Strip Scrabble. For each fifty points earned by a player, his or her competitor must remove one piece of clothing. The player with the most points, wearing the most articles of clothing wins. (Of course, that's debatable.)

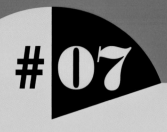

MORNING RING TOSS

Any time you've got a lot on your agenda (think weekday morning) and not much time to mess around first thing in the morning, opt for a cock ring. It temporarily creates more sensitive, intense, and hard erections. If you slip it on your lover as soon as he wakes in the morning while his cock is still hard or semihard, he'll be primed for high-speed action.

Estimated time: 3 minutes
What you'll need: a cock ring, kept on the bedside table; lubrication, also kept nearby; to be clear-headed and dexterous in the morning

THE PLAY BY PLAY

1. He's probably still half-asleep, but, girlfriends, you need to be bright-eyed and bushy-tailed. With a cock ring in hand, you have the chance to give him a wake-up call he won't forget.

2. Reach over and pick up the lube and the cock ring from the bedside table. Roll over onto your side and face your guy. While he's still groggy, lubricate his cock (which may be fully or partially erect) and balls, so the ring will slide on more comfortably.

3. Cock rings are usually worn around the base of the cock *and* the balls. You can put it on just his shaft (and by all means, experiment!), but it works best when secured around both his balls and his cock. This allows blood to flow into the erection, but not out of it, so hardness and sensitivity increase.

4. Try not to be nervous. A focused mind and steady hand will do the trick. First, pull the loose skin of his scrotum through the ring, then slide one testicle and then the other through. Finally, push his penis through.

5. For safety and pleasure, a cock ring needs to increase the size of the erection only slightly. If you notice more pronounced swelling, then the fit is too tight. In that case, take the cock ring off immediately.

6. Now that he's fully erect, you may want to tease the tip of his penis by licking or flicking with your finger. It will be highly sensitive.

7. When he's ready to put his hard, aroused cock inside you, release him from the ring and enjoy your morning balling.

8. No time to linger. Race to the shower!

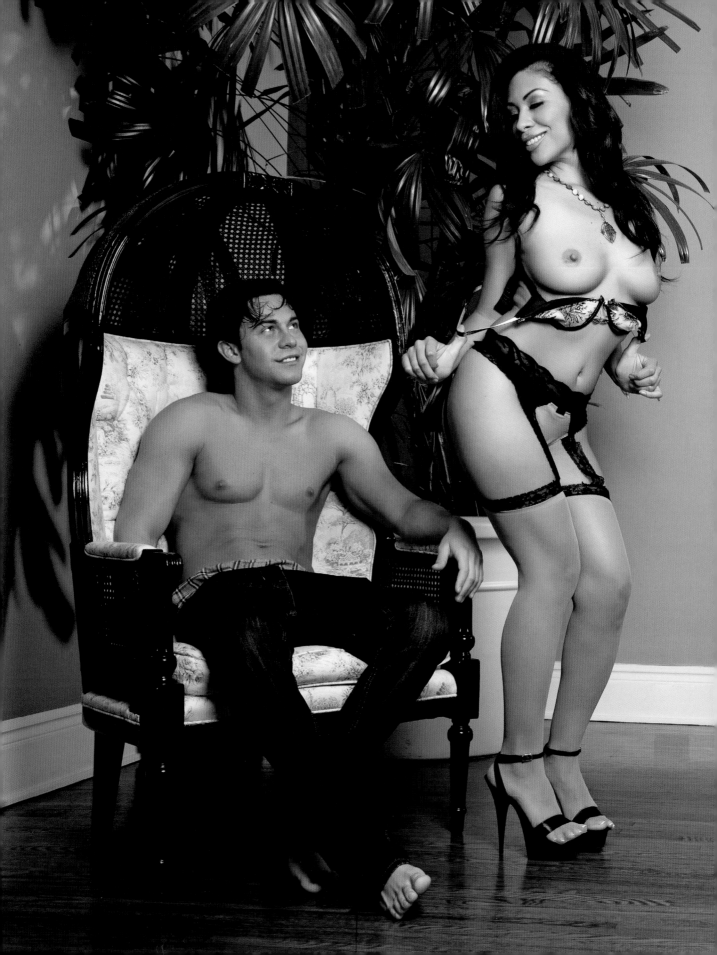

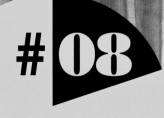

NAUGHTY NIGHT STRIPTEASE

This is the perfect scenario for that Friday night when the kids are away. It is also perfect because every man loves a striptease. It gets him hornier than all-get-out. And you can give him one without making a huge, time-consuming production out of it. After all, you're probably undressing for bed anyway.

Estimated time: 8–12 minutes
What you'll need: music, a scarf, sexy clothes that come off easily (e.g., skirt, blouse, stockings, garter belt, high heels), a chair

THE PLAY BY PLAY

1. Ladies, don't keep your intention a secret. Dim the lights and pat the edge of the bed with a come-hither attitude and coax him to sit right down and watch the show.

2. Turn on the music. It will help you keep the beat—but go for s-l-o-w, moody tunes. Remember, this is a striptease—emphasis on *tease*. You can use the following instructions as a guide, but you don't need to follow them step by step.

3. Start to unwind your scarf. Run it seductively through your hands, then over your shoulders and from side to side, arching your back at the same time. Use it as a blindfold, put it around his neck to draw him close—use your imagination!

4. Take off a piece of clothing very, very slowly. With your back to him, look over your shoulder. Shrug your shoulder up sexily so your blouse slides down in one motion. Turn around to face him, and *then* remove the blouse/jacket and drop it on the floor.

5. With your back to him, look over your shoulder. Unzip your skirt as slowly as possible, sticking your butt out and arching your back. The skirt should be off in one quick, smooth motion. Once it's on the floor, step out of it and leave it there.

6. Next, simply lift your leg up behind you, reach back, and use your hand to gracefully remove your high heels.

7. Now you're ready to slide off your stockings. Maintain eye contact while putting one leg up on a chair. Undo the garter belt first, then roll down the stockings using both hands, one on each side of your leg. Nice and slow. Keep rolling the stocking down until your hands are on your ankle. Once you've slipped the stocking off your heel, remove it from your foot with finger and thumb. You can use it as a prop to drape around his neck. Without pausing, unclip and fling your garter belt.

8. Face him and slowly shrug your bra straps down. Take it off slowly and drop it, with one arm covering your breasts.

9. Next, go for the payoff: your panties! Keep one leg in front of the other with your heel lifted. Put your hands (palms facing legs) completely inside the straps at the sides of your panties, lifting them up and away from your legs, then slide your hands and panties down your body. As your hands move down, your body follows. Step out one foot at a time.

10. Walk around for a moment in all your glory—then tackle him. He'll be more than ready.

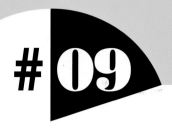

WE ALL CREAM FOR ICE CREAM

Ice cream is everyone's favorite dessert, so why not combine it with everyone's favorite naughty activity? Treat yourselves to a delectable cone that is more than just a scoopful of calories.

Estimated time: 5–7 minutes
What you'll need: ice cream cone (sugar), one scoop of soft but not melted ice cream, a towel, a kitchen chair

THE PLAY BY PLAY

1. First things first: You both agree this ice cream cone is for sexual pleasure.

2. Next, girlfriends, you grip an empty sugar (not waffle-style) cone in your hand while he pulls his still-soft penis out of his pants. Keep a towel within reach because this can be gooey but oh-so-worth-it.

3. Bite off a big piece of the cone's end and slip it on top of his still soft cock. Don't fret: He won't be Mr. Softee for long.

4. Now add the ice cream on top of the horizontal cone. Choose a smooth flavor that doesn't have nuts, fruit, or chunks of candy, and make sure the ice cream is soft enough that it doesn't crack the cone. How much fun is this?

5. Next, take your ever-lovin' time licking the ice cream until he's so hard that he breaks out of the cone. This shouldn't take long.

6. Gobble up the last drips and keep sucking until he's had a delicious climax.

7. Your turn? Guys, dip your tongue into the ice cream and explore your woman's pussy and clit with chilling success.

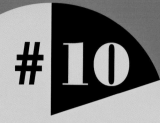

X-RATED BEDTIME STORY

Does your bedtime ritual involve propping yourselves against your pillows and delving into a book? If that's the case, try something new tonight by telling each other (and acting out) an erotic tale. Hint: Research shows women are aroused by stories where the male dominates. "She was all alone and defenseless when ... "

Estimated time: 10 minutes
What you'll need: a good imagination, handcuffs, blindfold

THE PLAY BY PLAY

1. When you first get into bed, snuggle up and agree on who is going to begin the tale of dangerous seduction. If you know you're both into playful bondage, acting out a good dungeon story might be the way to go.

2. Blindfold and bind your lady with handcuffs.

3. Ready guys? Begin reading (or come up with your own start): *It was a dark night when an armed guard brought Isabelle in handcuffs and blindfolds to the stranger's house. The door opened. "You have her, good! Bring her to me NOW," the stranger commanded in a deep threatening tone.*

4. Chime in now ladies, in your most alarmed voice: *No! No! What are you going to do to me?*

5. Guys, step into the stranger's character: *Bring her closer. I want to see how wet she is and if she's ready to be treated to pleasure and pain beyond her wildest dreams.*

6. Ladies, whimper and beg for mercy. *Oh, please, please, don't hurt me! Don't treat me like a slave.*

7. Let's take a break: Telling a bedtime story like this is a safe way to explore even your darkest fantasies, so don't hold back. The more personal and authentic, the more it will turn your partner on. *"Be quiet or I'll put a gag in your mouth,"* the stranger can threaten, or whatever else may turn you and your partner on.

8. Stay in character. Guys, finger her clit or just lay your palm over her mound to tease her as she whimpers. If she obeys to your commands and begins begging for your cock, pinch her nipples and tell her with sinister mocking *"All in good time."*

6. Keep the act going and tease until the pressure builds and must be released. Now unlock her handcuffs but keep the blindfold on; staying in the dark brings arousal to a whole new level.

6. Rock her world until the only word she can scream is your name, over and over again.

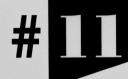

SURPRISE GREETING

Sex therapists say you can turn the element of surprise into instant foreplay. The next time you're dressing for a night on the town—*don't*. Stay naked and cover yourself with a coat, then stand by the door. Right before you're ready to leave the house make your big reveal.

Estimated time: 12 minutes
What you'll need: a cover-up coat, lube in your pocket

THE PLAY BY PLAY

1. If your lover man is like most guys and you're like most women, he's already hot under the collar because it seems like it's taking you forever to get ready for your night out. There he sits in the living room, twiddling his thumbs and watching *Family Guy*. Don't be tempted to let the pussy out of the bag by making your dressing time any shorter than usual.

2. When he's not looking, be sure to bring your best cover-up coat into the bedroom. Wrap it around your naked body. Now remain calm and casual and don't let him know you're naked when you walk out of the bedroom. Even if he asks to see what you're wearing, for at least another minute just offer a Cheshire grin.

3. As he opens the outside door, flash the big reveal. Guaranteed, he'll be shocked!

4. But don't stop there. Take the lead and go to the next level. Turns out men love women who take charge. According to one poll, men rate the sexual aggressiveness of their current partner as a 5. What do they really want? According to the poll, it's an 8. Give it to him—now.

5. Slowly and seductively strip him of his clothing, unbuttoning, unzipping, and pulling his pants down and off. Murmur words of appreciation.

6. Don't waste time getting to the bedroom. You can make love on the hallway floor. If you're in the mood to role-play, you might suggest he let you be the dominatrix. If he agrees, position your guy so he's lying on his back, one leg outstretched and the other bent, knee pointing upward. Make him do what you want by using a strong arm or a husky, take-no-prisoners voice.

7. Now take the lube out from your coat pocket and stroke it on his penis until he responds. Then straddle his body sideways with your back turned slightly to his face; hold on to his knee, and lower yourself onto his penis. In this pose, your stomach is almost touching his bent knee; use it for support and leverage as you rock back and forth, and up and down. The steady rocking motion primes you for the Big O.

8. Needless to say, you'll be thrilling him, too. For an added zing, wrap your hands around his legs and offer a titillating thigh massage at the same time.

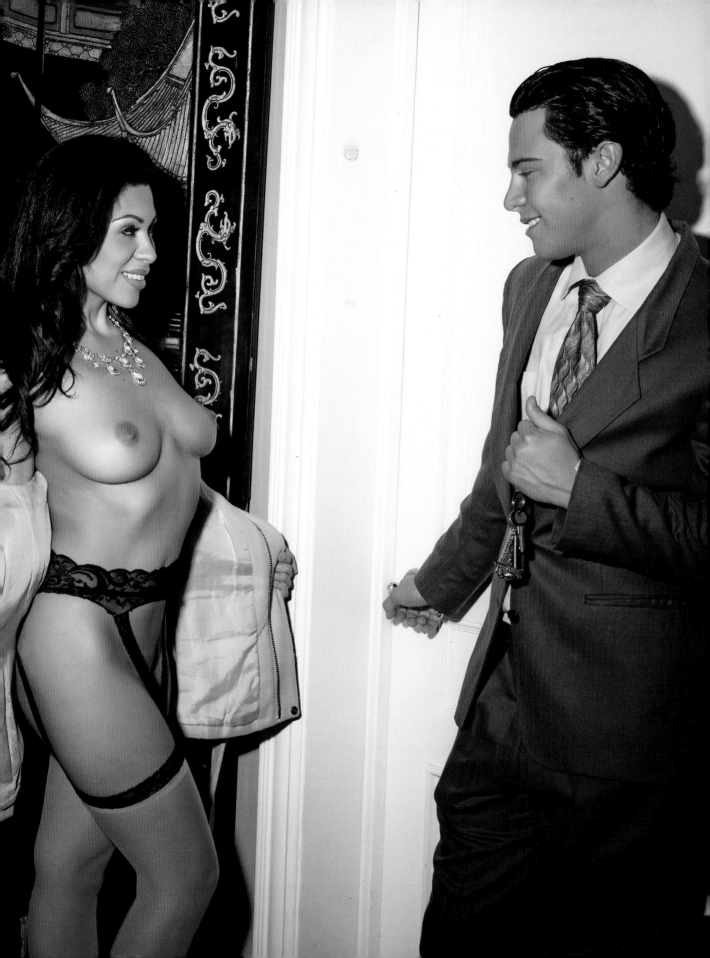

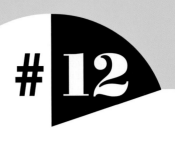

CAR KEY GROPING

The average person spends 55 minutes a day looking for misplaced items. That adds up to a total of almost 14 days a year just trying to find our stuff. Well, since you're hunting for the keys anyway, check out your partner's pocket—and hope you find what you're *really* looking for. Don't waste any precious time.

Estimated time: 5 minutes
What you'll need: lube (keep it in *your* pocket)

THE PLAY BY PLAY

1. "Darling, do you have my keys?" you coo. "I've looked all over for them."

2. Of course, he'll say no—but don't accept his answer. You need proof. "Just let me check," you say. Now slip your hand into his pocket and feel around.

3. Keep groping until you can feel his shaft. "Oops, what's this?" you wonder aloud. Move your fingers over and around his rod until you feel him responding. It will help if you nibble on his ear, breathe heavily, and moan with appreciation.

4. Once you sense a reaction, it's your cue to slip your hand out of his pocket, pull down his zipper, and start pumping. (Be sure to use lube first.)

5. Try the Clasping Hands Job. Place both hands around his penis, as if you were praying, and keep the motion going.

6. Remember to tighten the clasp of your hands during the upward strokes, especially on the tip of his penis.

7. *Ahhhhhh* ... What's this? Oh, it's the key to his climax.

TOOLING AROUND

If your man has a workshop or tool bench, chances are you'll find him spending his spare time there. But even do-it-yourselfers appreciate an occasional helping hand. Jerk him off in a way he'll never forget.

Estimated time: 10 minutes
What you'll need: a wrench, lube (keep it in your pocket)

THE PLAY BY PLAY

1. Got a handyman for a honey? Consider yourself lucky. Even though he might be concentrating on a home improvement project, there's an excellent chance he won't mind "screwing" around if you approach him in an irresistible way.

2. Slink up beside him and ask if you can interrupt for a moment. Use your most seductive voice. Remember, if he's in the middle of a project, you'll have to lure him away (or flash him). Put any sharp objects out of reach—except for the wrench. Grab it and slowly wave it in front of his fly giving him a sensual look.

3. As you gently move the wrench up and down his covered bulge, tell him how much a man who works with his hands turns you on. Then begin to talk about his attributes, concentrating on his beautiful, well-endowed, responsive cock. Give him an idea of what you mean by stroking the wrench playfully.

4. Now get on your knees. While at eye-level with his zipper, describe how good his penis will feel in your hands. Then unzip his pants. He'll expect you to put his cock in your hands, but hold off. Pick up the wrench and tap it ever-so-lightly against his shaft. Nothing like a little danger to get a handyman hard.

5. Once it has served its purpose, put the wrench on the floor and take his cock in your hands. Start to pump slowly and tell him you need to do some tightening up on him.

6. As you reach for the lube, talk about how you want him to come for you and where—on your face, stomach, breasts, etc.

7. Use a whole hand grip and lots of lube to "jack" him off. Imagine you're fitting that wrench around his shaft. You want to apply just the right pressure.

8. If you desire, lower his pants and under-wear and give anal stimulation a try. If he isn't against it, finger his anus a bit. The easiest and best way to produce the male orgasm is by prostate massage. The only way to do that is by sliding a well lubri-cated finger inside his anus. Not too deep, but an entire finger length (without pushing deeper) will do the trick.

9. This is the kind of handiwork you'll both appreciate. When he's satisfied to the max, hand him the wrench and tell him to get back on the job.

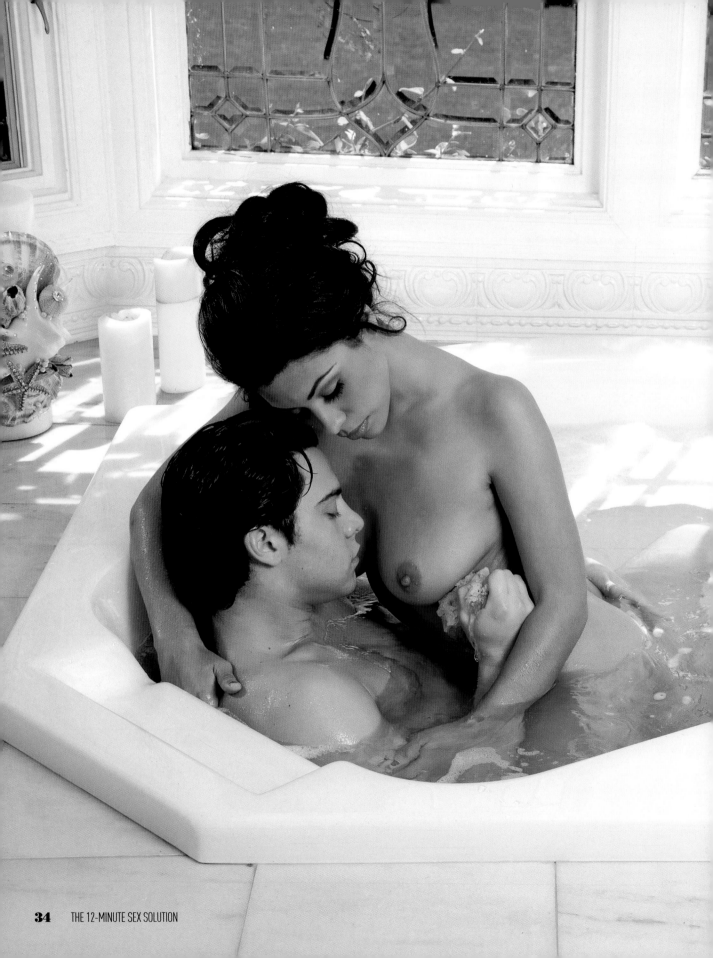

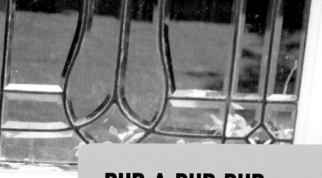

#14

RUB-A-DUB-DUB

It's a slow Sunday and the kids are still with their grandparents. Why not get your juices going with a water fight? The bathroom might be a squeaky clean locale, but your goal is spend your time getting as filthy as possible. Still, you don't want to go over your head with desire—first agree on a safe word and always pay attention.

Estimated time: 12 minutes
What you'll need: a water gun, a sponge or washcloth, a bath mat, a scratchy loofah, a safe word

THE PLAY BY PLAY

1. Your man is a bandit who's just bombarded you in the bathroom. He holds a loaded water gun pointed in your direction and commands you to "Strip naked and fill the tub *or else* ..."

2. You comply. "Now get in," he says in his most threatening voice, "And be still ... Not a word out of you!"

3. Guys, strip fast but keep the gun handy and don't take your eyes off your "victim." If your lady moves, tell her you're going to shoot. If she doesn't believe you and she shifts in the tub, tell her to spread her legs over the bath rim and spray her thighs in a tantalizing way. "I'm not kidding!" you say as you wave your other hardening hot rod—the one between your legs.

4. Now kneel on the floor and dampen the loofah with bathwater. "You've been very dirty," tell her in a threatening voice. "I'm going to have to punish you."

5. Demand your lady turn around and raise her butt. Give her a few smarting slaps with the wet loofah. When she's good and aroused and her butt is rosy, join her in the tub.

6. Get on the bottom and instruct her to straddle your lap (facing your feet) and slowly lower her onto your penis. This will give you a good view of her shiny wet and spanked derriere.

7. Be forceful and tell her to ride you until you say she can stop. Keep smacking her ass and telling her you'll only show mercy if the job is well done.

8. Ladies, lean forward so you're resting on your palms. In this position he can hold onto your butt or thighs and ride 'em straight out of this world.

9. Guys, when you're close to orgasm, instruct her to turn back around so you can show her your softer side and reward her for high-caliber work. As you reach orgasm together, run the sponge down her body and tell her she was the only jewel you were really after anyway.

03

CHORE-PLAY
A Whole New Way of Looking at Your Dryer and Other Appliances

Is there anyone out there who looks forward to vacuuming the rug, cleaning the oven, or taking out the trash? Well, probably not—until now. In this chapter, you'll get the PLAY BY PLAY on how to enjoy skillful and passionate lovemaking even while doing humdrum housework. Chores that may have triggered a bout of resentment can suddenly take on a whole new pleasurable dimension.

For instance, the laundry room is for getting clothes clean, right? But you can also use it to get down and dirty, since heat and vibration amp up orgasmic sensations. Or when you're working in your home office, why not keep a vibrator in the desk drawer and pop it inside your panties or boxers while you're balancing the checkbook? Waiting for the pasta water to boil? It's a perfect time for steamy phone sex.

In this chapter, you'll discover multitasking inspiration as well as hands-on activities to ensure your love life is always intimate and action-packed, even when duty calls.

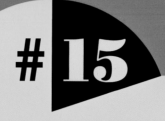

"ON HOLD" HAND JOB

Okay, name one thing more annoying than being put on hold and waiting... waiting...waiting...waiting...for an operator to take your call. It's the perfect opportunity to have sex. You have one hand free, right?

Estimated time: suggested wait time of at least 5 minutes
What you'll need: lube, patience, an ear to the phone ... just in case

THE PLAY BY PLAY

1. With one hand holding the phone, the other one is free to work magic on your guy's cock. If you don't have lubrication nearby, use your saliva.

2. Beckon your man over and tell him you're bored with *just* holding for the operator. Can he do you a favor and stand by? Then surprise him by tugging at his zipper and letting him know what you really want to be holding: his cock.

3. After you've pulled his shaft from his underwear and it's out in the open, lube or wet your hand with saliva.

4. Remember the preferred direction for movement during a hand job is toward his body so that he's experiencing the same sort of movement from your hand as he would from intercourse.

5. The pressure of the grip is important. Imagine holding a peeled banana just lightly enough so you don't mush it.

6. Are you still holding for the operator? For a change, add this motion: Starting in the middle of his shaft, work your hand in a twisting motion from base to tip and back to the middle again. (Imagine ever so lightly wringing out a wet cloth—similar idea here.) If he's not in love with this move, he'll let you know.

7. Start slowly and ramp up the speed as he gets harder. Continue pumping.

8. Should the operator pick up the line before he's reached a climax, keep your priorities in order and continue the hand job. Now who's the smooth operator?

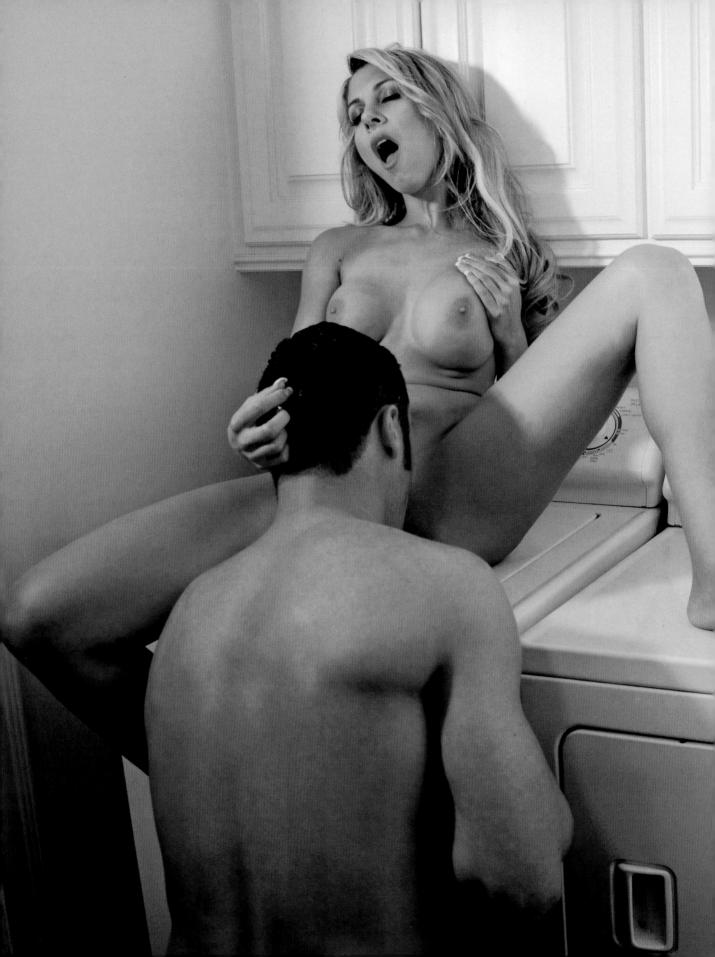

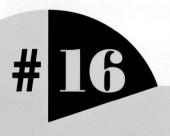

SPIN-CYCLE SEX

As a mover and shaker, you don't want to waste your day *just* doing the laundry. So when the washing machine is running, opt to hop on top and have sex while it's on the spin cycle. Try to do it in the nude because the machine's vibrations will excite your bare bodies. And you'll be able to save time by washing your clothes while making love.

Estimated time: 12 minutes—although orgasm by intercourse sometimes requires more time
What you'll need: a washer and dryer in a private location, the willingness to sit bare on an appliance, wash-and-wear outfits

THE PLAY BY PLAY

1. Each of you should strip down to your birthday suits, tossing your clothing into the laundry with the rest of the wash.

2. Guys, you'll want to sit your nude lady on the edge of the machine with her legs bent and feet on your shoulders. As the machine pulsates, bend or kneel and give her delectable oral stimulation. The key here is to make sure that the clitoral hood is out of the way. The pulsations of the cycle will help bring blood to her pelvic area and enhance her stimulation and excitement.

3. Next, turn your woman around and have her lie face down on top of the washing machine; keep your feet flat on the floor. Stand facing her from behind, spread her legs with your hands, and enter her vagina. She should be plenty wet after you've licked her clit.

4. This position is not the same as anal sex. If your lady needs reassurance, let her know you're simply using the rear-entry position that allows for both deep penetration and vigorous pushing, which is especially exciting while the machine is vibrating. In this position, guys can reach the clitoris easily, and his hands are free to caress her body at the same time.

5. As the washer reaches its spin cycle, lean forward so that your thighs press against her. The vibrations will rock through both your bodies.

6. If you have time to spare, hang out afterward for the heat of the dry cycle. Then dress one another in your freshly washed and warm clothes.

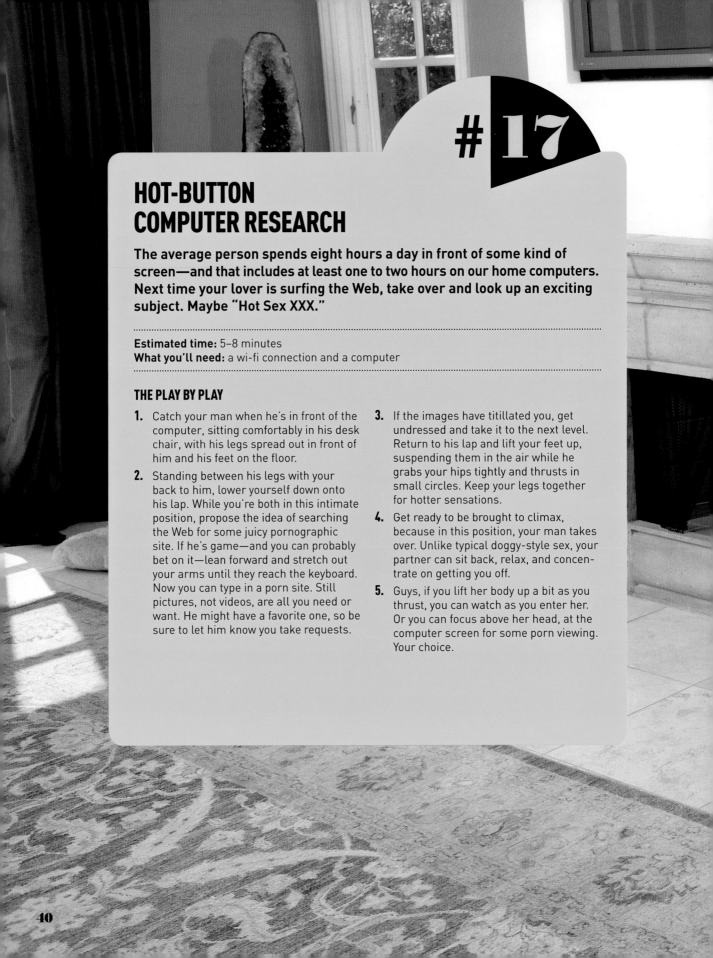

#17

HOT-BUTTON COMPUTER RESEARCH

The average person spends eight hours a day in front of some kind of screen—and that includes at least one to two hours on our home computers. Next time your lover is surfing the Web, take over and look up an exciting subject. Maybe "Hot Sex XXX."

Estimated time: 5–8 minutes
What you'll need: a wi-fi connection and a computer

THE PLAY BY PLAY

1. Catch your man when he's in front of the computer, sitting comfortably in his desk chair, with his legs spread out in front of him and his feet on the floor.

2. Standing between his legs with your back to him, lower yourself down onto his lap. While you're both in this intimate position, propose the idea of searching the Web for some juicy pornographic site. If he's game—and you can probably bet on it—lean forward and stretch out your arms until they reach the keyboard. Now you can type in a porn site. Still pictures, not videos, are all you need or want. He might have a favorite one, so be sure to let him know you take requests.

3. If the images have titillated you, get undressed and take it to the next level. Return to his lap and lift your feet up, suspending them in the air while he grabs your hips tightly and thrusts in small circles. Keep your legs together for hotter sensations.

4. Get ready to be brought to climax, because in this position, your man takes over. Unlike typical doggy-style sex, your partner can sit back, relax, and concentrate on getting you off.

5. Guys, if you lift her body up a bit as you thrust, you can watch as you enter her. Or you can focus above her head, at the computer screen for some porn viewing. Your choice.

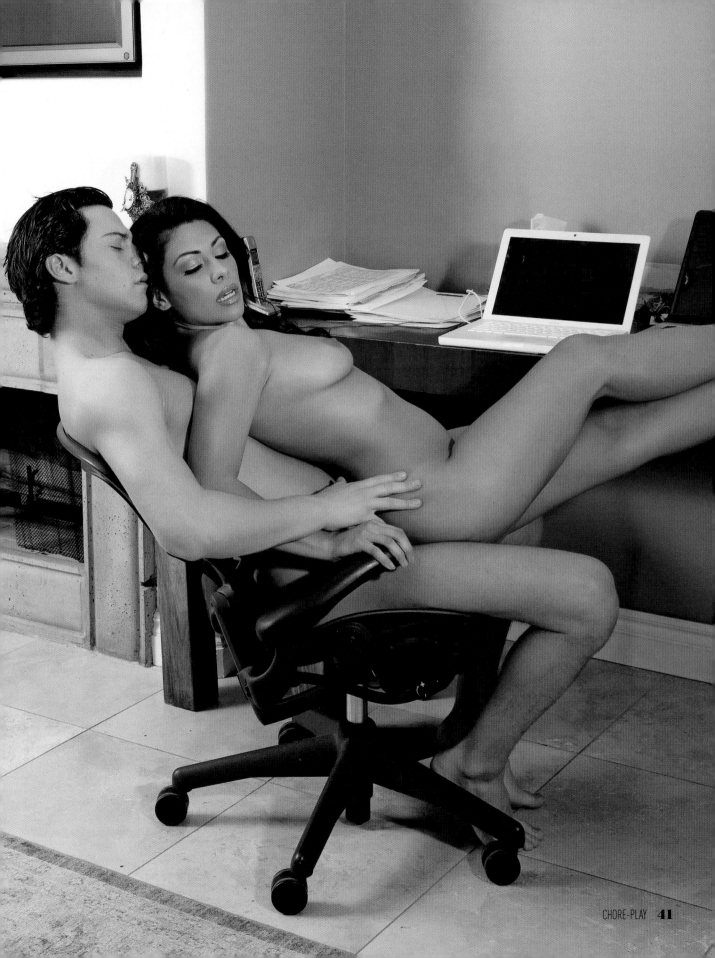

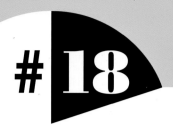

DISHWASHING DIVERSION

Studies show people spend more time in the kitchen than in any other room in their house. In fact, it's been described by sociologists as the "heart center." That's why the kitchen is where you'll find the most opportunities to save time and "multi-task." Pick a night when everyone else is out (or upstairs doing their homework) and begin at the sink.

....

Estimated time: 5–7 minutes
What you'll need: lube, a wet spoon or spatula, a damp cloth, the surprise factor

....

THE PLAY BY PLAY

1. Guys, when your partner is washing dishes, sneak up on her from behind.

2. Slip your hands around her waist. Kiss the back of her neck and gently play with her breasts.

3. If she's not complaining and you sense she's responding to your playfulness with equal enthusiasm, lift her skirt or lower her pants and pull her panties down.

4. Massage her mound with one hand and before you turn off the faucet with the other hand, reach for a wash cloth or dish towel and drench it. Smack her behind with the wet rag. Now turn off the faucet (you want to prevent flooding) and rub her butt playfully.

5. Reach into the soapy sink and pull out a spoon or spatula. Tease her by running it up and down her inner thighs. Tap lightly on her rear again. Just when she thinks you're going to smack her again, retreat and toss the utensil back in the sink.

6. Now make up for being such a bully. Get on your knees, turn her around to face you, spread her thighs and lubricate her with your tongue and free hand. Pick up the damp cloth again and rub it on her ass and over her breasts.

7. While you're giving her unforgettable oral sex continue to smack her silly until she sinks to her knees and returns the favor.

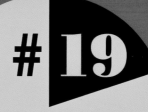

 # 19

DIRTY WINDOW WASHING

You probably don't wash the windows too often, but next time you do, it's an ideal chance to explore the exhibitionist in you. If you like the idea of possibly being seen during sex, then this is *clearly* the setting for you.

Estimated time: 5–8 minutes
What you'll need: window-washing props, a wide window ledge or seat, chutzpah

THE PLAY BY PLAY

1. Tempt your man to play along by leaning against the window ledge provocatively. Not wearing panties is a good start; chances are you'll snag his attention.

2. Once he's standing in front of you ready to explore you down there, take the lead and yank down his zipper and pull out his penis and testicles. You needn't be too gentle.

3. Now stand up and beckon him to take a seat by patting the windowsill so his back is toward the great outdoors. Slide onto your knees and remind him that the neighbors may be watching,

4. In the position you're in, he'll be expecting you to slip his penis into your mouth, but instead lead his hand to his cock. At the same time, start rubbing your clitoris with your palm. Some guys get self-conscious about masturbating in front of a lover

because when they touch themselves they connect with their own private fantasy world, so he might be hesitant to touch his works. You can encourage him by taking his hand in yours and guiding his fingers to his shaft. Meanwhile, continue pleasuring yourself with your other hand.

5. Guys learn early in their lives the most effective way to get themselves off and most never waiver from their tried-and-true approach—which is fine. Try not to interrupt his train of thought by contributing to his technique. Just let him do his own thing.

6. Meanwhile, he may be busy watching you while you reach climax. Imagining the neighbors could be doing the same will automatically add new potency to your self-pleasing.

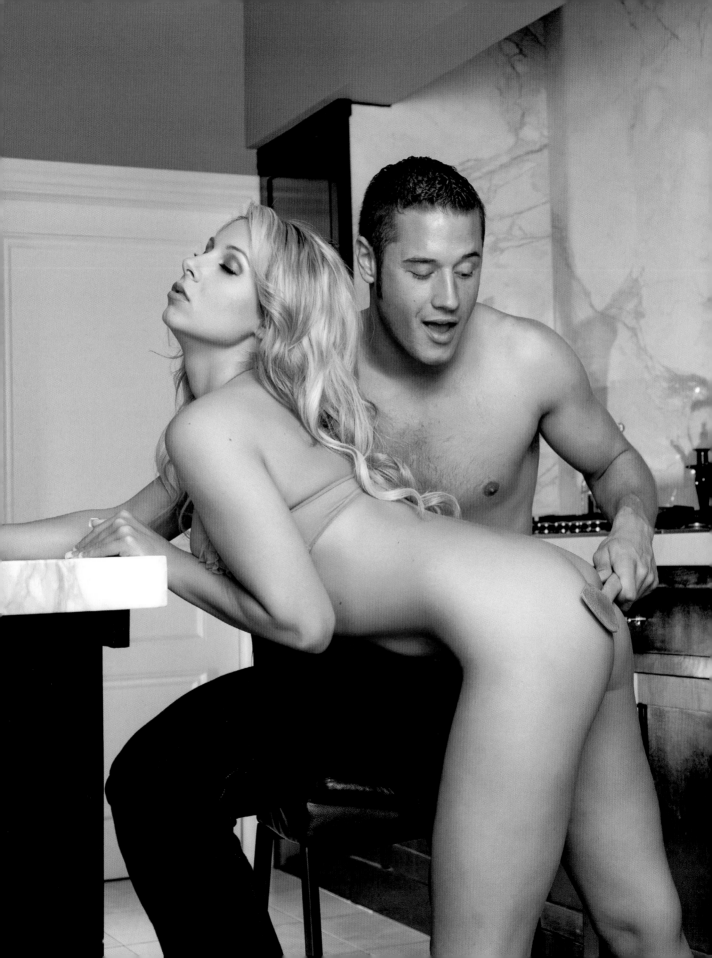

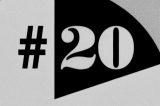

SPANKING APPETIZERS

Hungry and just hanging around until the order arrives? There's no reason to waste another hungry minute. Enjoy a good spanking session. Spanking is sexy and satisfying! Studies show a majority of women have fantasies about being spanked, and most men find spanking a woman to be a strong sexual turn-on.

Estimated time: 5–10 minutes
What you'll need: a steady hand or wooden spoon, a cushion (optional)

THE PLAY BY PLAY

1. What makes a spanking session perfect while you're waiting for a delivery to arrive is that it's a given you're both hungry. Aching to be satisfied is an excellent way to begin the session.

2. Remember, playful spanking is never about brute force. It's just another way to focus the mind and body so orgasm can be achieved. If you want to get technical, here's how it works: The physiological process of sexual arousal demands that before orgasm occurs, blood must be collected and kept in the genitals and nearby areas. Spanking creates just such a physiological response because the stinging skin causes blood to collect in the bottom and the nearby genitals, accomplishing manually what caresses and kisses do psychologically.

3. A terrific way to offer your lover the kind of spanking she really deserves is to give it to her over your knee or on a cushion so her bottom is kept propped up and supported. This will cause her butt to squirm from the sting, simultaneously resulting in her rubbing her clitoris on your supporting knee, the cushion, etc.

4. The feeling of surrender or submission is an important part of a woman's sexual response; many women need to give themselves permission to feel sexual.

5. The best spanking technique is to slightly cup your palm with your fingers pressed together. This creates a smacking sound and reddens the skin, all without causing excessive pain. If she seems to be unmoved by such spanks, give her a few with a flat palm and relaxed-but-spread fingers—those sting the most. Keep it up until she squirms or responds in other ways, such as little yelps or whimpers. You can also alternate with quick and light whacks with a wooden spoon.

6. Use a slow tempo with an irregular rhythm. The moments of anticipation between each stroke add to the tension.

7. Every guy who knows his partner's signs of arousal can judge when the time is right to shift her from the spanking position onto your erect shaft. Unless, of course, the doorbell rings. If so, it's one more hearty slap before it's time to satisfy your *culinary* appetites.

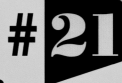

#21

CUPCAKE-COOLING CUNNILINGUS

The recipe says you have to wait until the cupcakes cool—at least 10 minutes—before you can have a taste. Take advantage of the waiting time by engaging in another treat: fingering. By the way, studies show a combination of oral and finger sex results in more orgasms than any other sexual practice.

Estimated time: 6 minutes
What you'll need: pillows for your knees, lube, a vibrating toy (optional), a mixing spoon

THE PLAY BY PLAY

1. With the sweet aroma of cupcakes wafting through the kitchen, thank your baker by offering a different kind of treat. Explain that she's worked so hard, you want to say thank you. Then guide her to a kitchen chair and pull her pants down or her skirt up.

2. Place two pillows under your knees and get comfortable.

3. Spread her legs and take her clit into your mouth and gently suck on it.

4. Suck or nibble her labia.

5. When she's good and excited, generously lube your finger and add penetration. If you'd like to make the experience even more intense, lube up a vibrating toy and gently insert it into her vagina. If you're using your finger, move it in and out using short but firm strokes. If you're opting for the vibrator, you can let it linger by her clit before insertion. Rule of thumb: Always be gentle when using a toy.

6. Now that her arousal is peaking, it's an excellent time to offer her a tasty distraction. Take the batter-covered mixing spoon and offer her a taste. When it's wiped clean, give her a light but smarting smack on her butt. This will immediately bring her arousal rate up again.

7. Now that she's hotter than those cupcakes in the oven, go back to your finger, put your mouth on her clitoris, and lick her while you penetrate her. This won't do it for all women, but many love the experience of clitoral stimulation and finger penetration.

8. Keep a steady pace and avoid stopping.

9. You'll start to see the signs when she's getting ready to go over the top—her moans, her thighs pressing against your head, her body arching, her hands tightening on your head …

10. Even though your sweetie will need a few more minutes to cool off, the cupcakes are ready. Why not feed her one?

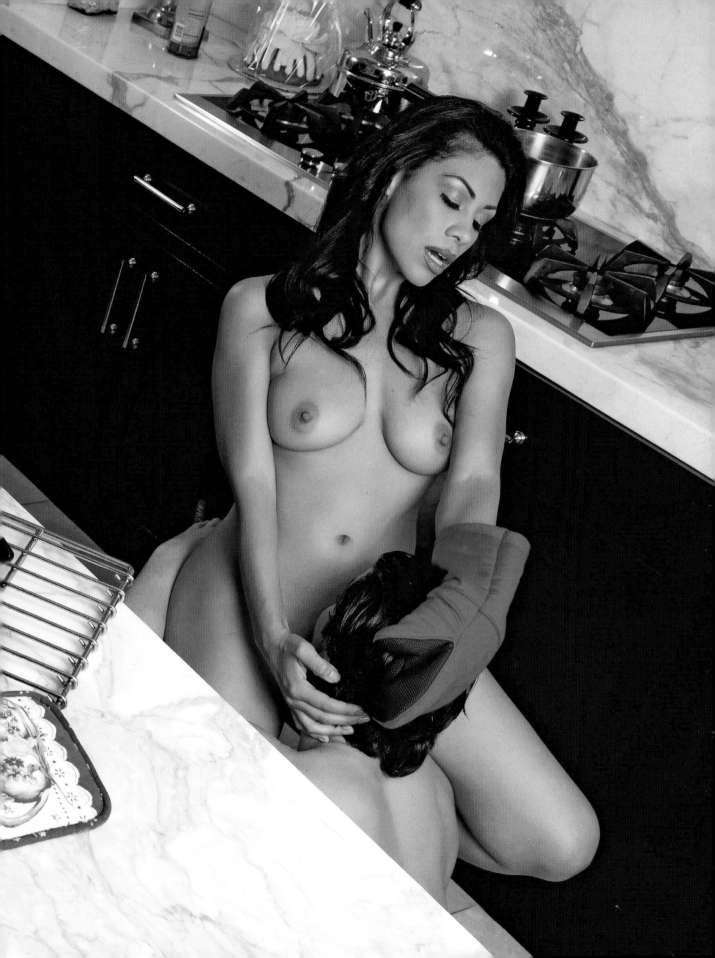

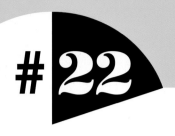

 # 22

BETWEEN-COURSES FELLATIO

If you're having a dinner party at your house and your guests are happily conversing with each other after the appetizer, excuse yourselves to go in the kitchen and prepare the main course. Explain that the dish needs a few last-minute touches, and tell your partner you need his help. Here's your chance to give him a surprise appetizer he won't forget. Work quickly before guests suspect foul play.

Estimated time: 5 minutes—that's all you've got before the guests wonder what's going on, so use your time wisely

What you'll need: an edible lube if you've got it handy, or lots of saliva

THE PLAY BY PLAY

1. Since your partner thinks he's really needed in the kitchen and therefore isn't expecting a blow job, you'll probably be dealing with a soft penis at first (although some guys get erect with the surprise factor). In any case, you don't have to wait for it to get hard. Give him a deep kiss on his mouth, then slide down, unzip, and pull out his works.

2. You'll both have to be pretty quiet. No problem for you because you'll have something in your mouth. Lick it. You can sweeten things up by applying an edible lube, or if there's something sweet and gooey on the kitchen counter from meal prep, like honey or maple syrup, smear his cock with it.

3. Slide your lips over your teeth for smooth sailing.

4. You can do more wonderful stuff with your mouth than just suck. Mix it up by licking the sensitive underside of the shaft, the nerve-ending-loaded head of the penis, and the testicles, and then blow softly on the moistened areas. The combination of sensations will feel incredible.

5. Next, grip your guy's cock around the base and slide your hand up and down, hand job style, in tandem with your mouth. (Some guys like a tight squeeze, while others do not, so check in.) You can cover a lot of the shaft this way without worrying about taking the whole cock in your mouth. Concentrate on the super-sensitive head and suck as hard or softly as you and your partner like.

6. Chances are your partner will climax before the guests start wondering what's going on. But keep your ears tuned to the dining area. If you hear a lull in the conversation or guests questioning what you're doing in there, you might have to finish up what you started after they leave and while the dishes are soaking.

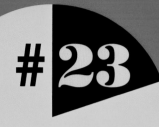

NAIL-DRYING BONDAGE

As every beauty-conscious girl knows, waiting for your nails to dry is completely ho-hum. B-o-r-i-n-g. Since you have to remain immobile anyway, make the most out of your limitation. This simple S&M play gives your man all the power.

Estimated time: 10–12 minutes
What you'll need: lube; handcuffs, scarves, or rope; a bed with posts or a headboard

THE PLAY BY PLAY

1. The submissive person (that would be you with the wet nails) is positioned like an eagle with spread wings. This can be done lying down or standing. Since bondage is being used, it's easier to opt for the prone position.

2. If you're lying on a bed, your hands should remain curled up toward the headboard and your feet toward the opposite end, legs spread. You can be tied down with ropes or scarves, or handcuffed. Tell your partner to be careful to bind your wrists so your hands can remain facing upward to protect your sticky nails.

3. If you're not already wet with anticipation, your partner should apply a suitable amount of lube. He needn't be too gentle about it, either.

4. Now that you're snugly bound and wet, your master mounts you, giving him the feeling of complete power and you the sense of utter and total vulnerability. You cannot get much more open and vulnerable than being spread-eagle and having *everything* exposed.

5. You will need to basically stay still, except for wiggling and squirming. This guarantees your nails will dry unharmed and you'll both feel the intensity of this playful S&M position.

6. Even though you're just playing, be safe and follow the general rules of bondage, including having a safe word. As long as you play within the rules, research shows the psychological turn-on of bondage quickens arousal and leads to satisfying, mind-blowing orgasms.

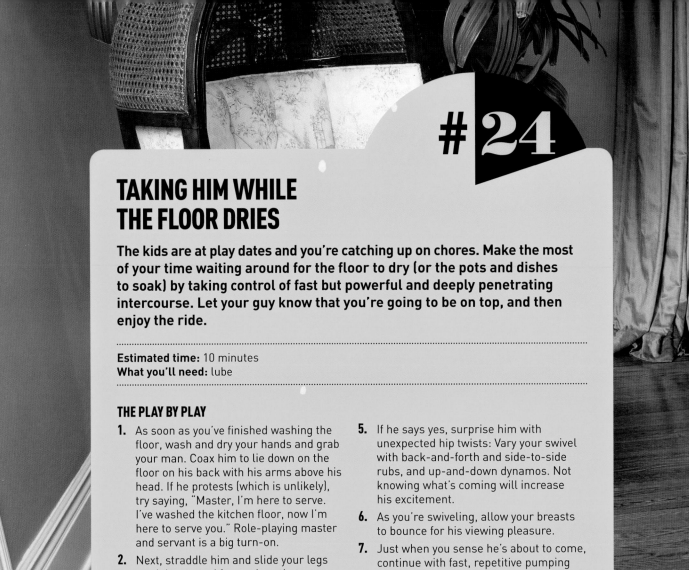

TAKING HIM WHILE THE FLOOR DRIES

The kids are at play dates and you're catching up on chores. Make the most of your time waiting around for the floor to dry (or the pots and dishes to soak) by taking control of fast but powerful and deeply penetrating intercourse. Let your guy know that you're going to be on top, and then enjoy the ride.

Estimated time: 10 minutes
What you'll need: lube

THE PLAY BY PLAY

1. As soon as you've finished washing the floor, wash and dry your hands and grab your man. Coax him to lie down on the floor on his back with his arms above his head. If he protests (which is unlikely), try saying, "Master, I'm here to serve. I've washed the kitchen floor, now I'm here to serve you." Role-playing master and servant is a big turn-on.

2. Next, straddle him and slide your legs straight out and forward, so that your feet are on either side of his shoulders.

3. Then be bold and hold his shins or push on the floor for leverage and start swiveling your hips in figure-eight motions so you're moving his penis around inside like you would move a joystick for a video game.

4. Just like a joystick, you control the speed, direction, and overall activity level. Take your time because the floor is drying and certainly doesn't need your attention. Ask your master if he likes what you're doing.

5. If he says yes, surprise him with unexpected hip twists: Vary your swivel with back-and-forth and side-to-side rubs, and up-and-down dynamos. Not knowing what's coming will increase his excitement.

6. As you're swiveling, allow your breasts to bounce for his viewing pleasure.

7. Just when you sense he's about to come, continue with fast, repetitive pumping actions.

8. If you can't climax with him in this position (which is often the case), allow your clitoris to rest against his prone thigh and hump until you cum.

9. The floor should be dry by now—but you won't be.

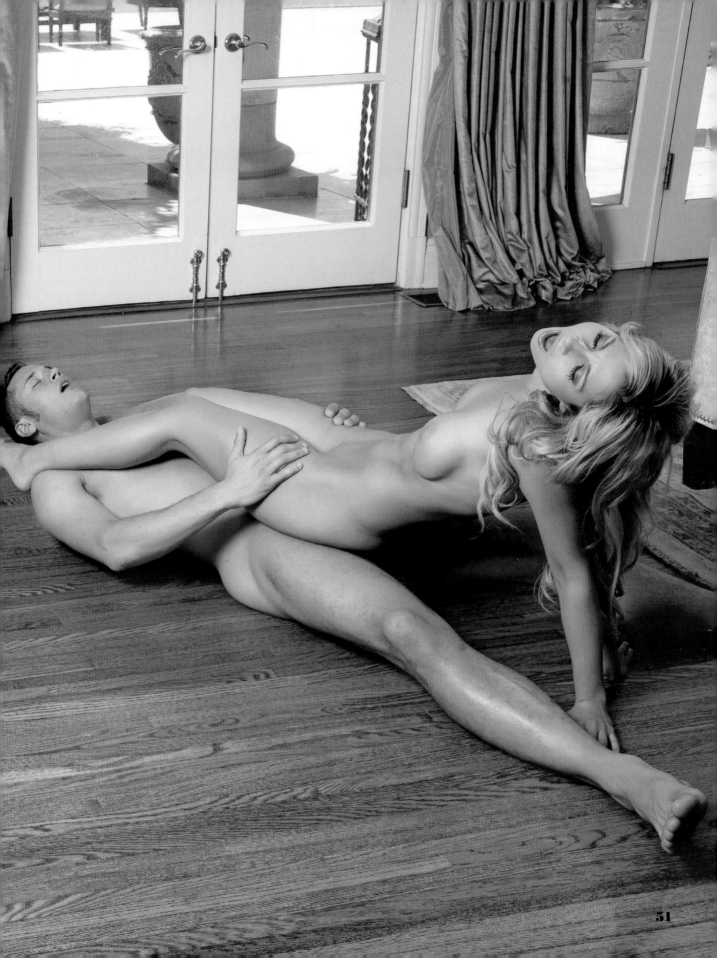

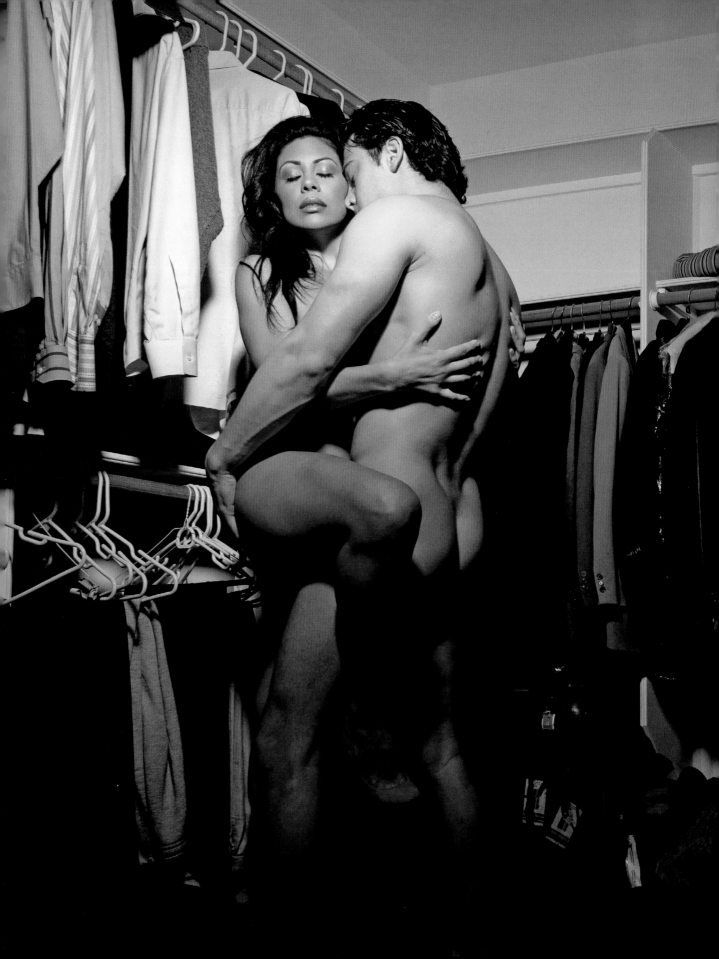

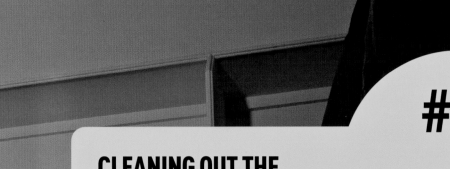

CLEANING OUT THE CLUTTER CLUTCH

It's as good a time as any to clean out your closets and donate bags of clothing, shoes, and purses to charity. Look! Now there's plenty of empty closet space! What are you waiting for? Closets are confining, private, and dark and provide an illusion of safety—all these elements heighten stand-up sex's lust factor.

Estimated time: 8–12 minutes
What you'll need: a little floor and wall space; no claustrophobia; lube; a belt, tie, or scarf

THE PLAY BY PLAY

1. You've both been working hard and in close quarters while getting rid of all that stuff you don't need. But don't close the door on your good deed just yet. Try enjoying the fruits of your labor. Begin with a full-body press.

2. Stand-up sex works best when you're close to the same height, so if your guy's got a few inches on you (or vice versa), stand on a filled carton or something sturdy enough to hold your weight (not a pile of clothes). You want to be eye-to-eye.

3. Now that you're facing, hold each other in a loose embrace.

4. Guys, bend your knees to slightly lower yourself so you can enter her, and then slowly rise. If she's dry, be sure to have lube handy.

5. Ladies, you'll have to lean back slightly so his pelvic bone presses against your clitoris on each thrust.

6. If you crave deeper penetration, try standing on one leg and hooking the other around his. Guys, hold on to her suspended thigh to help support you. Your lady won't have the opportunity for much movement (which can heighten arousal!), but you can add subtle shifts in motion by rocking her back and forth.

7. You're in the closet, so use what's available. Reach for a belt, tie, or scarf and wrap it around your woman's waist to bind her close to you and increase the intensity and control.

8. Ladies, for even more vertical variety, stand with your back to your guy, bend at the waist, and have him enter you from behind. Belts, ties, and scarves are especially handy in this position to help with balance. Not only will he be able to achieve deeper penetration, but also one hand will be free to titillate the rest of you until you both make the closet shake.

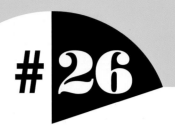

#26

BREAKFAST BONANZA

Forget instant oatmeal. Opt for old fashioned steel-cut oats, which are high in B vitamins, calcium, and protein, and contain more fiber than a bran muffin. Best of all, they take between 20 and 30 minutes to cook, so while the oatmeal pot is simmering and the kids are still in bed, you'll have plenty of time to work side-by-side with your mate to build up an appetite.

Estimated time: up to 12 minutes
What you'll need: kitchen table or counter, a pot of slow-cooking oatmeal, raw oatmeal, soft stick of butter, milk, maple syrup, wet dishtowel

THE PLAY BY PLAY

1. Once the oatmeal starts simmering, give it a full stir, turn it down to low, and organize the props you'll need (see above). Be sure to keep them within reach of the pot.

2. Next strip naked. Ladies, position yourself so you're sitting on top of the counter or kitchen table.

3. In this instance, the chef will also be the diner, so decide who wants to take charge. If it's very early and you're both groggy, leave it up to your man. He's likely to rise to the occasion faster.

4. Gals, spread your legs wide and be ready to receive. Guys, begin with the stick of butter. Run it along the inside of your lover's thighs, massaging and licking as you go. Be sure the butter is room temperature, not hard and cold!

5. To make her blood rise, add a little friction by creating a patty of raw oatmeal and milk in your palm, then rubbing it from her thighs to her knees, to her calves, and down to her feet. Pay special attention the erogenous soles of her feet. Suck her toes if you're so inclined.

6. Now "clean" her up with a warm dishtowel. But don't leave her untouched for a second. Once you're finished, fling the used towel to the side and reach for the maple syrup. Pour the syrup into your mouth and hold it there until you transfer it to her pussy.

7. Get licking. The sweet and sticky syrup will work her into a state. After she's reached a sweet orgasm, pour syrup onto your cock and masturbate until you reach a climax.

8. Perfect timing. The oatmeal should be about ready. Wash up and dig in. Oh, don't forget to add (fresh) butter and syrup. Remind you of something?

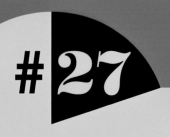

FRESH LAUNDRY

Need help folding the freshly laundered sheets? Call your guy over and request a hand. As he walks closer, double the warm sheet—and tackle him lustily to the ground.

Estimated time: 7–12 minutes
What you'll need: massage oil, a pile of clean laundry

THE PLAY BY PLAY

1. Good ploy! You've got him where you want him; don't waste another minute. Take even more control and help him strip off all his clothes. Tell him resistance is futile.

2. Reach over to the pile of warm, clean, white laundry and grab two towels. Bind his hands together with one and his feet with another.

3. If he complains, take even more power and slip a pillow case over his head. Leave it loose so he can breathe and tell him not to utter a word. Be commanding—he'll be happy to oblige!

4. Now you've got him where you want him. It's your turn to undress, but do it quietly so he doesn't know what's happening.

5. Rub his body generously with the massage oil you have handy. Start with his arms and legs, torso and feet, but save his loins for last. Don't worry about making a mess! You've got everything covered with sheets and towels and you can wash them again, anyway.

6. When you see he's aroused, roll on top of him and squirm. Feel his oiled body and his rising cock.

7. When you sense he might explode, pull yourself off. Straddle his torso and lick his balls and shaft and then go at him in earnest with a rhythmic sucking action.

8. Right before he comes, pull back and slide back on top of him, putting his hard cock inside you. You're both likely to climax simultaneously with a juicy explosion.

9. Accept the fact that your laundry will need to be rewashed—but hey, if you're still in dominatrix mode, make your grateful man take care of the chore!

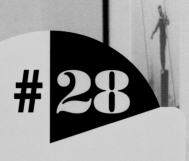

WORK IT IN YOUR HOME OFFICE

Millions of people work from their homes at least occasionally, which means there are plenty of chances to engage in the classic role-play of boss–secretary.

Estimated time: 10 minutes or less
What you'll need: a sturdy swivel chair, preferably leather; a lock on the door

THE PLAY BY PLAY

1. Ladies, get in the mood for role-playing. Put on your slinkiest skirt and tightest sweater and knock on your hard-worker's door. "Mr. VanBoss, do you need anthing?" you ask in your formal, subservient voice. But don't wait for an answer—just walk in clutching a pad and pen.

2. Have a seat across from the boss's desk and for a few brief seconds, slide your legs slightly apart and give him a quick view of your pantyless crotch, à la Sharon Stone.

3. Then get up, and keep your gaze on him while you walk around his chair and begin to massage his neck.

4. In your huskiest "screw me" voice, say, "You need to relax, Mr. VanBoss. You've been working too *hard*." These words should get his mind going in the right direction.

5. Next, spin the chair around and straddle him so he's powerless to move.

6. Squirm, bite his ear, whisper dirty possibilities, and keep it up until you feel him get bigger. Then slide down to the floor and get on your knees.

7. Pull his zipper down with your teeth and expose his cock. "Why, Mr. VanBoss, I didn't realize you were so *big*," you might say. As you know, it's always a good idea to compliment the boss.

8. A long, slow lick along the underside of his shaft from base to top will emphasize his length. Use the flat part of your tongue to encircle his shaft.

9. When you want him to climax, concentrate on the frenulum and coronal ridge where the glans and shaft meet. Flick and circle it with the tip of your tongue in a consistent rhythm. Keep going until you prove to him who is really the boss.

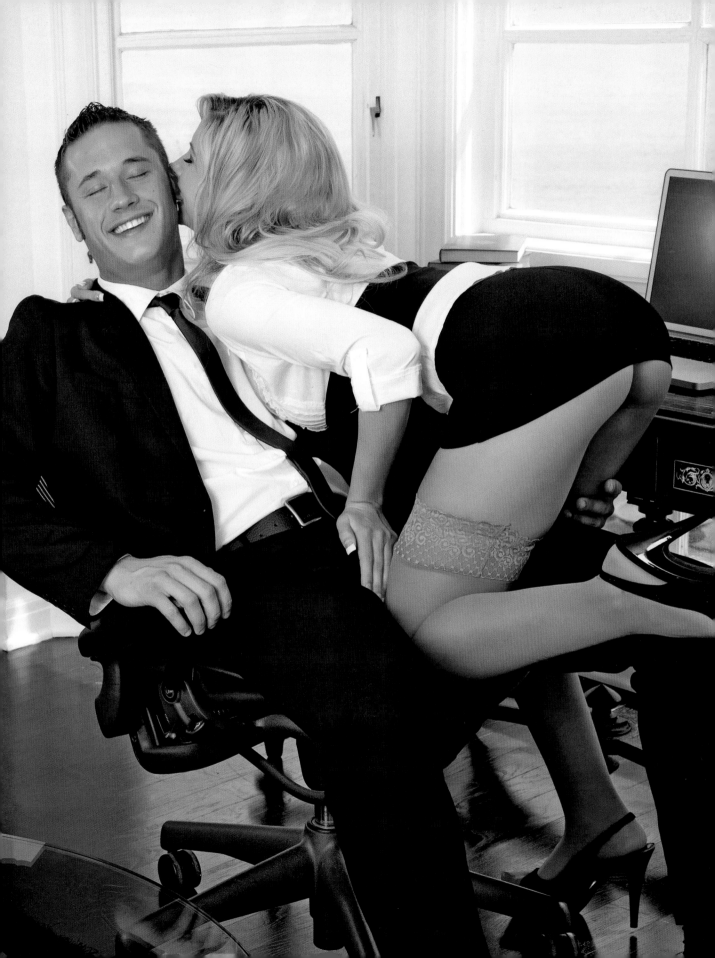

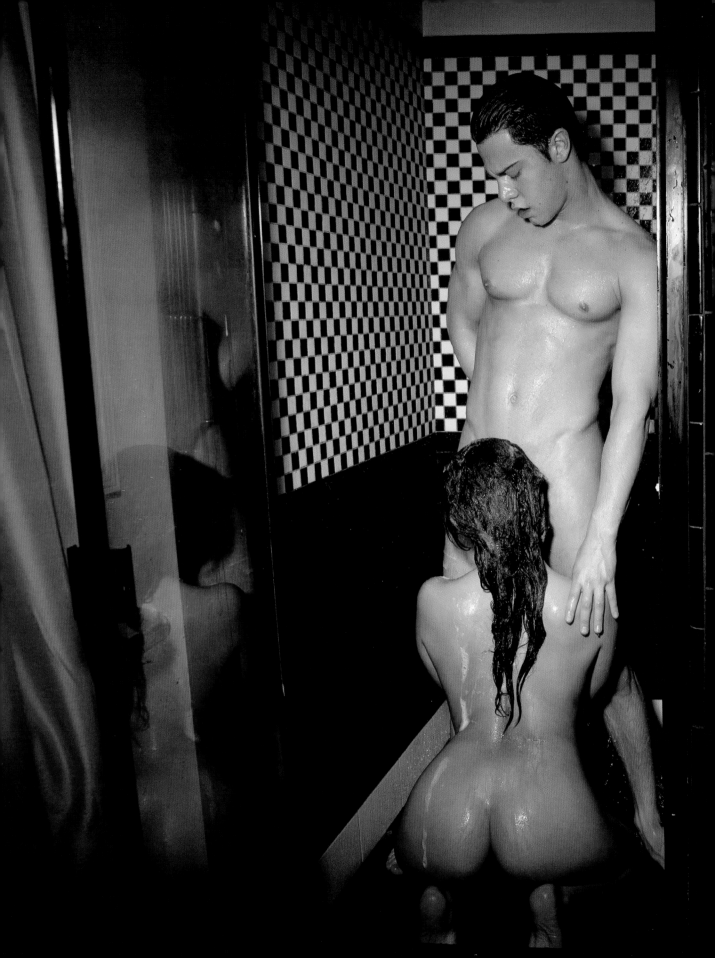

SHAMPOO AND *BLOW* DRY

Most of us wash our hair at least three times a week, if not daily. Why not offer a fast, hair-raising blow job while your guy is lathering up? You won't have to interrupt your usual routine, morning or night, and even better, if you time it right, the kids will be asleep.

Estimated time: 5 minutes or less
What you'll need: non-irritating shampoo (kids' shampoo is ideal), a large bath towel, hair dryer

THE PLAY BY PLAY

1. While your guy is washing his hair, go ahead and join him in the shower. You can count on the water being just the right temp so step right in.

2. As he's lathering his mane, get on your knees and concentrate on his pubic hair. Slowly drip the shampoo down his mound.

3. Move the palm of your hand slowly in circles, creating foam and excitement. You'll be tempted to do something about his rising cock, but don't. Let him get hornier before you satisfy his craving.

4. When his pubes are washed clean and smell sensational, cup water in your hand, and rinse slowly. Let the water pour over his cock, sensually tantalizing it. Again, you'll both want the satisfaction now, but resist.

5. Stroke his shaft while you put his balls in your mouth, licking and sucking and getting him ready for the grand finale.

6. Now's the time to move on to his rock-hard cock. Avoid being in a position where your face is getting bombarded with the relentless spray of the water. You'll want to be able to breathe freely.

7. Put his eager wet cock in your mouth and suck rhythmically.

8. For added fun, if you have a removable showerhead, pull it down and let it rain on his parade (or yours). Then resume sucking until he comes.

9. When he's out of the shower, continue paying exclusive attention to his pubic area. Use a hair dryer on warm *not hot* to fluff him up. That's one happy and groomed cock!

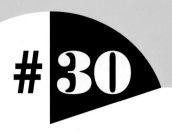

 # 30

MAKEUP SEX

Not the kind that says "I'm sorry" but the kind you do while you're putting on lipstick and mascara. Face it, mirrors are notoriously sexy. And watching yourself as you do it makes it doubly hot.

Estimated time: 7 minutes or less
What you'll need: lube, a mirror, lipstick

THE PLAY BY PLAY

1. Guys, catch your beauty by surprise in the morning while she's putting on her makeup. There's nothing like a little fright to get a lady hot. Don't hesitate; grab her from behind and coax her hands free of any beauty products. If the kids are still home, lock the door—"makeup" is for adults only, after all.

2. She'll be able to look at you in the mirror's reflection. Return her gaze with lust in your eyes so there's no mistaking what you're there for. You don't have to say much, just help her lean slightly against the sink, keeping a steady gaze on her eyes. Then put her hands on the sink to guarantee she'll get the support she's going to need.

3. Don't take your gaze off each other. It's said that the eyes are the window to our souls, and the mirror image cinches the connection.

4. Hold her hips, grab the lube that's on the counter, give her a good smearing, and enter her from behind. Be prepared for a squeal of delight. Standing gives more thrusting power and allows for deep penetration, and her body is angled so that her G-spot will be stimulated by the thrust of your penis.

5. For added erotica, reach for her lipstick and swirl it around her nipples, turning them into pink or red bullets.

6. Depending on how far bent over you are and how fast you're thrusting, your testicles will slap against her vagina, which can be very exciting. For added pleasure, offer her clitoral stimulation while you're thrusting. Remember to keep your gaze steady on your reflection in the mirror as the heat and desire increase. Let those moans of pleasure bounce off the bathroom walls!

7. After you've both reached orgasm, it's back to makeup. No doubt her mascara will need repair. But since you're still feeling the intimate connection, ask if she'd like you to apply her lipstick. Yes or no, turn her around and offer a warm kiss of appreciation.

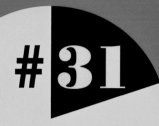

BEAT THE CLOCK

Oh, those fashionably late guests. While you're waiting for them to show, grab this timely opportunity. Urgency can trigger an explosive encounter and not knowing when they'll arrive makes sex even riskier—and hotter.

Estimated time: 10 minutes
What you'll need: coat or jacket to put under your knees

THE PLAY BY PLAY

1. To add heightened suspense to your last-minute lovemaking, first leave the front door open so guests can come in at their leisure. If you want to add even more danger, play music. This way even when they arrive, you won't be totally certain they're there.

2. A few minutes before the party is set to begin, retreat to the hall closet for your quick-and-dirty romp.

3. Set down a soft jacket or coat to protect sensitive knees. Strip down.

4. Each of you should now kneel on one knee (the opposite knee of your partner), and face each other, with the foot of your other leg planted on the floor. Inch closer to each other until your genitals are joined. This is a little like a teeter-totter, but with the heat turned up! Lean forward on your planted foot, enter her, and then rock back and forth as you get into the groove.

5. Keep in mind that guests could be right outside your door, so if either of you moans or gasps, the other must stifle it gently with their palm.

6. Even though there won't be a lot of in-and-out action (perfect for the confines of a closet), the slow torso-to-torso grind provides great clitoral contact as you each ascent to climax. Rocking back and forth in this position also keeps you as closely connected as two lovers can be.

7. Remember, it's easy to get lost in this trancelike position; if you want a heads up to pull your clothes on, keep one ear open to the door just in case the guests arrive *unfashionably* on time. (And if they do, wait until they've walked into another room before covertly slipping out of your hiding spot—they'll be none the wiser!)

TAKE OUT THE TRASH TACKLE

There's nothing more sexy than a man who takes out the trash (especially without being asked). Here's your chance to make the most of this chore's erotic potential!

Estimated time: 3–5 minutes
What you'll need: your best poker face, a tucked-away corner of your garage or house, lube

THE PLAY BY PLAY

1. Guys, claim you need a little help from your lady carrying out the trash (but be sure to stick some lube in your back pocket beforehand). If she's not convinced, tell her you think you may have thrown out an old photo of the two of you by accident and really need to find it. By doing this, you are showing both your sensitive side and your desire for her to be your partner in crime, which will make her feel not only desired but *wanted*. Cue the flying sparks!

2. When your lady arrives to help you in your search, sling your arm around her shoulder and lead her to a secluded part of the building or house. Admit your initial request for help was just a ploy, but you do really need her for some behind-the-fence debauchery. If you are up for role-playing, feel free to start pretending you're two high-schoolers again, sneaking away for a passionate rendezvous after school. For many women, talking your way into a sexual fantasy is a huge turn-on and will get you revved up in no time. Make yourself the captain of the football team and her the prom queen, or even just two shy kids with big crushes on each other.

3. Lean against the wall and turn her so her back is facing you. Kiss her neck and whisper words of desire.

4. Generously lube her up, and enter her as you would in standing rear entry—but lift her up by the hips and have her grip your waist with her legs. You'll be in a position similar to the wheelbarrow races you played in school, except this is even more fun.

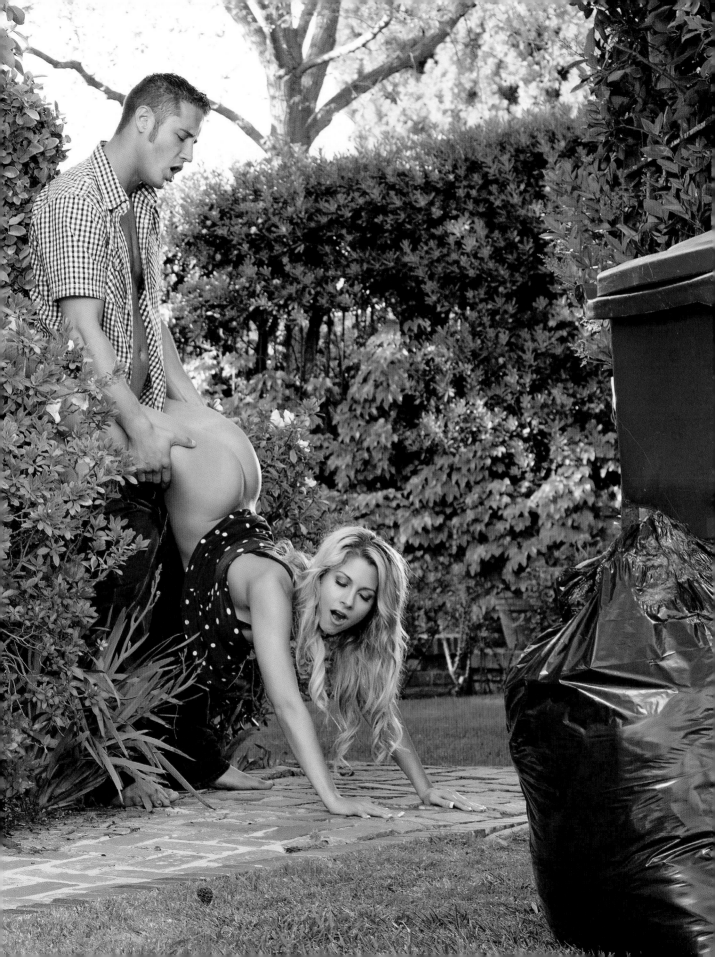

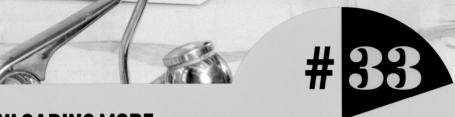

#33

UNLOADING MORE THAN THE DISHES

You put them in, you take them out. We're talking about dishes here, but of course you can imagine the same with certain body parts. So while you're waiting for the dishwasher buzzer to sound, use the warmth of the drying cycle, or steam through the door, to offer even more heat—and a memorable way to dish out an orgasm.

Estimated time: 12 minutes (the average dishwasher has a 15-minute dry cycle)
What you'll need: a dishwasher, lube, a mat, a warm spoon

THE PLAY BY PLAY

1. Be prepared. When the dishwasher is about to enter its dry cycle, place a mat in front of it and grab your honey. Strip down.

2. Guys, open the door for a second and let the steam out to warm up the area. At the same time, reach inside and pull out a hot spoon. CAUTION: Be careful not to burn yourself. A plastic spoon or spatula may be your safest bet.

3. Now FAST, shut the door, press the cycle back on and sit back against the dishwasher with your legs spread out on the floor.

4. Draw your lady on top of your cock and start to stroke her with the spoon, going up and down her back and down to her bum. Whisper dirty tidbits in her ear. Accuse her of being naughty and deserving a spanking.

5. Strike her playfully. When you feel her getting juicier, add a little more pleasure and reach for the lube. Put a copious amount on your finger and slip it into her pussy to join your cock.

6. Try to synchronize your orgasms with the sound of the all-finished dishwasher buzzer. If she can't get there in time and the buzzer does ring, keep talking dirty and don't break the momentum. Roll from this position into man- or woman-on-top (still on the floor) to encourage her climax.

7. Once your sexy cycle is complete, head to the showers for a double-duty rinse-and-dry of your own.

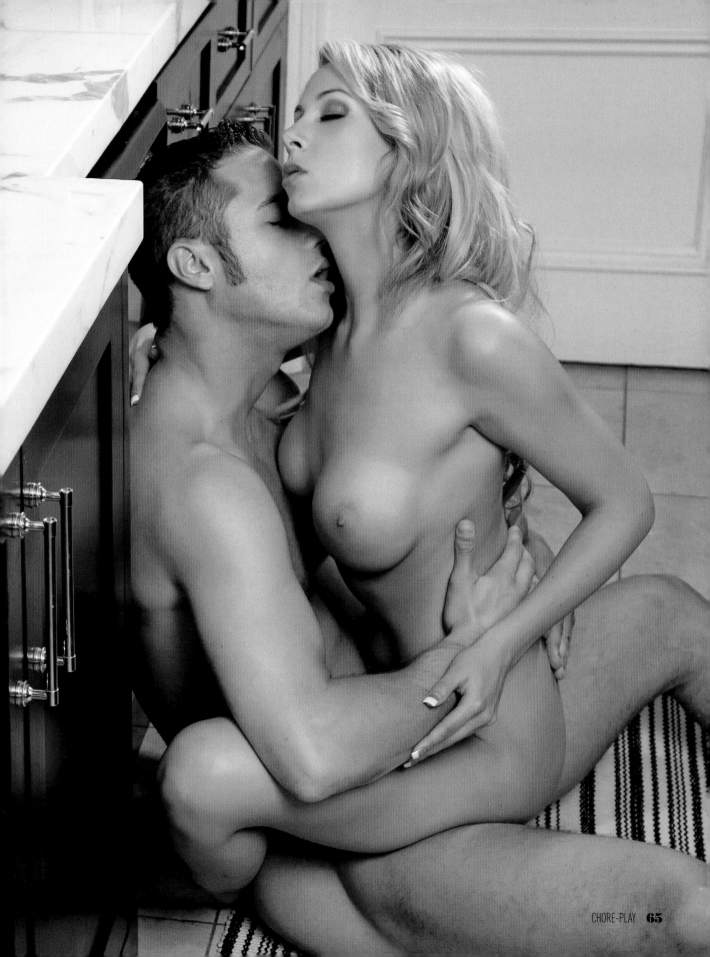

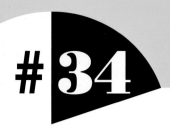

#34

BRINGING EGGS TO A HARD BOIL

You're under the gun with a schedule that can't budge. No worries. In the time it takes to boil eggs for breakfast, you will jolt your lady awake with this _eggcellent_ technique.

Estimated time: 5 minutes
What you'll need: an uncooked egg, lube, a mat or towel

THE PLAY BY PLAY

1. While your short-order cook is standing over the stove concentrating on the boiling water, grab a raw egg and sneak up on her from behind. Keep the egg hidden from view.

2. Kiss her neck and coax her to lay on the mat or towel you've put on the kitchen floor. She might protest but remember you're a man on mission: You're there to bring your lady to orgasm. Convince her with sweet talk and guarantee that you won't let the eggs over-boil.

3. Once she's prone, place the egg precariously on her stomach, letting her know she can't move or the egg will break. This creates an imaginary restraint as hot as a frying egg on a summertime sidewalk. Take advantage of the heat. With your lubed index finger, gently probe her luscious vaginal lips and the area inside her honeypot and all around it. If she squirms, remind her of the egg balancing on her belly.

4. Since you're just using one hand, the other is free to pleasure her nipples or run up and down her body. Once she's close to orgasm, you may want to remove the egg from her stomach, since she won't be able to control that sort of twitching or shaking.

5. Your short order cook will probably be too weak-kneed afterward to do anything but swoon, so continue to be a knight in shining armor. Help her stand, wash your hands and prepare a breakfast fit for a princess. The eggs will be timed just right!

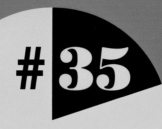

 # 35

SHAVING TIPS

May we suggest again that busy couples combine beautification with sexual satisfaction? Do it by shaving each other's pubes. Nothing says "hot" like a trimmed bush. It makes oral sex that much more exciting and so much tidier!

Estimated time: 5–8 minutes
What you'll need: scissors, electric trimmer or shaver (*no* razor blades!), a bed (because you won't be using soap, shaving cream, or water)

THE PLAY BY PLAY

1. Ladies, think *Steel Magnolias*, but instead of working on a sistah's hairdo, get down and do your man. While fondling his cock lovingly, take the electric shaver in hand and trim his pubes. Be creative! You can give him a boy's Brazilian or just neaten the area, or if your guy has hair to spare, create a design. The shaver's vibration and your undivided attention are guaranteed to get him hard.

2. Finish off your handiwork with either a hand or a blow job. With his pubes trimmed he'll appear bigger than ever.

3. Guys, resist the urge to snooze after you've been so fully satisfied. It's your turn to be creative. Just running the vibrating shaver over her pussy should do the job of encouraging natural lubrication. Take advantage of her gooey pussy by fingering her clit or going for a pearl-diving expedition. If the latter is your choice, you may come up for air with some errant hairs in your mouth. Just spit them out.

4. Since you're both on the bed, if you still haven't climaxed, 69 is another option for the freshly shorn.

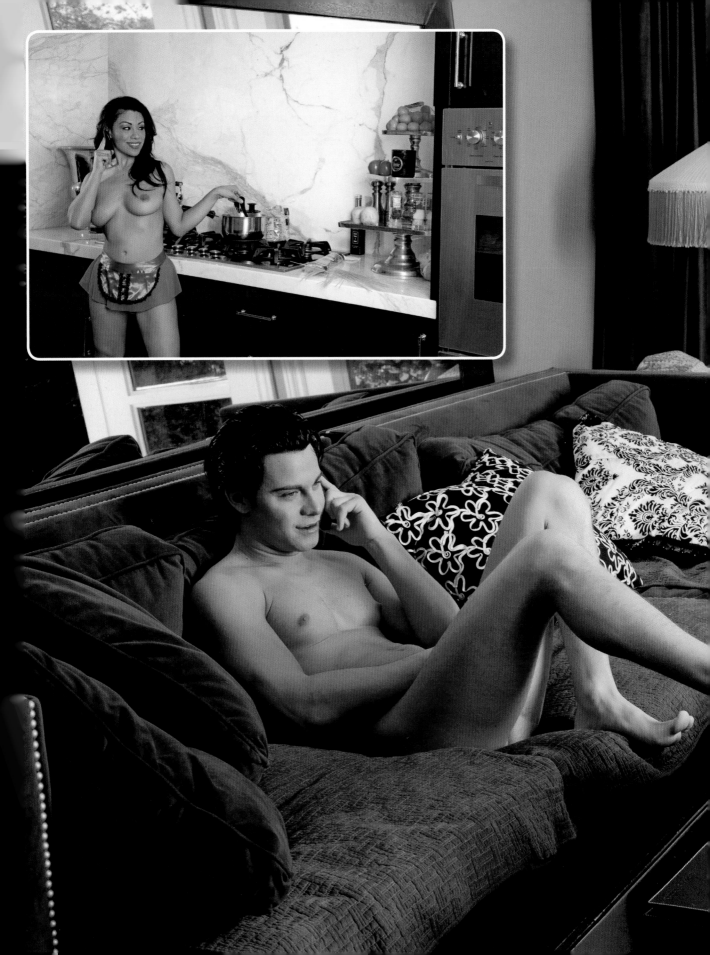

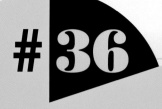

COOKING WITH PHONE SEX

After marking off your mile-long to-do list, of course you're too busy to prepare a five-star meal. Who needs it? A simple plate of pasta will be yummy. Even better, during the time it takes to bring the water to a boil, you can offer heart-pounding phone sex.

Estimated time: 10–12 minutes
What you'll need: a phone, preferably with a hands-free headset; another mobile phone; dinner in progress

THE PLAY BY PLAY

1. Let your guy know he's off the hook and doesn't have to help with dinner, but tell him you want to talk about something important and explain that it will be easier if you have the conversation over the phone. If he balks and wonders why you can't just talk things over in the kitchen, be creative. Tell him it's something so embarrassing that you'd rather tell him over the phone.

2. When he agrees, ask him to go in the bedroom and leave his cell phone on. You'll call in a minute. He might as well just make himself comfortable and wait on the bed.

3. Once he's out of the kitchen, plug in the headset to free up your hands and avoid a neck cramp. Now call your partner.

4. When he answers, in your sexiest whisper, say something like, "Oh, there you are. I've been thinking about you all day." Before he has a chance to respond ...

5. Begin a slow, relaxed, breathy conversation. To build up sexual tension, ask about his day and tell him about yours in a soft, sexy voice.

6. Gradually slip into steamy talk. Tell him, in detail, just how and why you missed him during the day. Describe the parts of his body that you admire the most, adding, "Just thinking about you makes me wet."

7. Tell him what you would want him to do to you, and ask him what he would like to do to you or like you to do to him in turn. Be flexible. Let the conversation lead itself. You don't have to stick to a fixed script. The point is to stay seductive—and connected. Dead air can dampen the mood, so fill in the blanks with heavy breathing, moaning, or simply whispering his name or a term of endearment.

8. Now tell him you want him to climax and coax him to pleasure himself. Ask him to describe what he's doing in detail. In response, breathe audibly and continue to encourage his actions. If possible, pleasure yourself at the same time. (You'll have to be safely away from any hot pots.)

9. When he climaxes, moan along with him. And after his breathing has returned to normal, tell him it's time for dinner. There's an embrace, a plate of pasta, and glass of wine waiting for him.

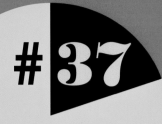

MORNING GROOMING WITH A HELPING HAND

You can only do this if your man spends a decent amount of time primping in front of the bathroom mirror. Encourage him to continue with his personal care while you whack him off.

Estimated time: 4–5 minutes
What you'll need: lube, shaving cream or lotion, a towel or bath mat, an eager groomer

THE PLAY BY PLAY

1. Who doesn't love a man who takes pride in his appearance? You can reward him for his expert grooming by using this technique, which mimics how he masturbates. He'll find it super easy to get aroused.

2. Smear your hands with some nearby shaving cream or lotion, and then kneel behind him (on a towel or bath mat) and stroke his thighs upward toward his cock.

3. Next, get some lube. (You don't want to use shaving cream or lotion here because it may sting.) Hold his cock at the base, and slowly start to move up and down the shaft with both hands. Don't be stingy with the lube.

4. Build up a smooth rhythm and keep your hands in contact with him at all times. Guys like to know if you have lost even a second of interest. If he looks down, encourage him instead to just keep looking at his handsome reflection in the mirror. It will help him stay focused and turn up the sensation of masturbation.

5. When you reach the tip of his penis, cup your fist over the head as if you're unscrewing a jar. Chances are good this is the way your man brings himself to orgasm. So continue the motion until he pops.

6. Grooming doesn't stop here; lick him clean if you're in the mood, or use a warm, damp cloth to tidy up.

04

GETTING FROM HERE TO THERE
The Best Ways to Go into Overdrive

Think about cars, and what comes to mind? Speed, power, and a sense of amazing freedom! That's why automobiles are perfect for fast-sex getaways. Car washes, service stations, junk-food drive-thrus, or just parking on the street can mean a killer blow job. Even while traveling alone, you can use a hands-free phone to talk dirty to your partner or masturbate with one hand; of course, keep your eyes on the road. Planes, trains, ferries, and buses are also tickets to ride your partner.

But don't put the brakes on there. Expand your desires to risky sexual encounters in the great outdoors. By taking sex out of the bedroom and into the fresh air, the world is literally your playground. Nature makes us feel alive and at one with our bodies and souls. Since much of our modern life is confined to small spaces, couples can break away and express themselves fully with outdoor thrills. Not to mention that the tension of being discovered is a way to bring you closer to your lover.

In this chapter, you'll learn how to let your desires loose whenever you get the chance, whether in the car, outside, or riding an elevator. Feel free to tune into your basic instincts, and don't forget to keep a blanket handy just in case you feel like getting down and naughty while on the go.

BACK STAIRS BOOGIE

There are two good reasons for climbing: First, it's terrific exercise; second, it's great for your sex life. Screwing on the stairs is best with this two-step position when it's peppered with imagination. So while the kids are sleeping, take it to the stairs!

Estimated time: 3–6 minutes
What you'll need: lube, easy-access outfits, out-of-the-way stairwell

THE PLAY BY PLAY

1. First, make sure you don't hear a peep out of the little ones. Then head for the stairs. You can certainly keep the lights dimmed.

2. There's no need to disrobe for your step-up adventure. Merely lift your skirt or robe while he unzips his pants.

3. To position yourselves perfectly, sit on the stair with your legs spread apart while your guy kneels two steps below.

4. Stair sex works best with role playing so get into the act by keeping a sexy conversation going. For example, pretend your man is a stranger meeting you on the back steps of a building and forcing you to have sex. (Keep the lube handy so

he can generously apply it to your pussy before he takes you with all his might.) Whimper quietly so you won't be discovered.

5. This is fast, take-no-prisoners inter-course. Stairs support even the most enthusiastic thrusts. As he "forcibly" enters you, he'll have to lean on his hands for leverage while thrusting.

6. Vigorous in-and-out movements will create carnal current that will hit your nether regions, boosting stimulation. But still—try to fight him off. If you can't resist, a good playful slap on the cheek of this bold stranger after the ecstatic deed is done will be well-deserved.

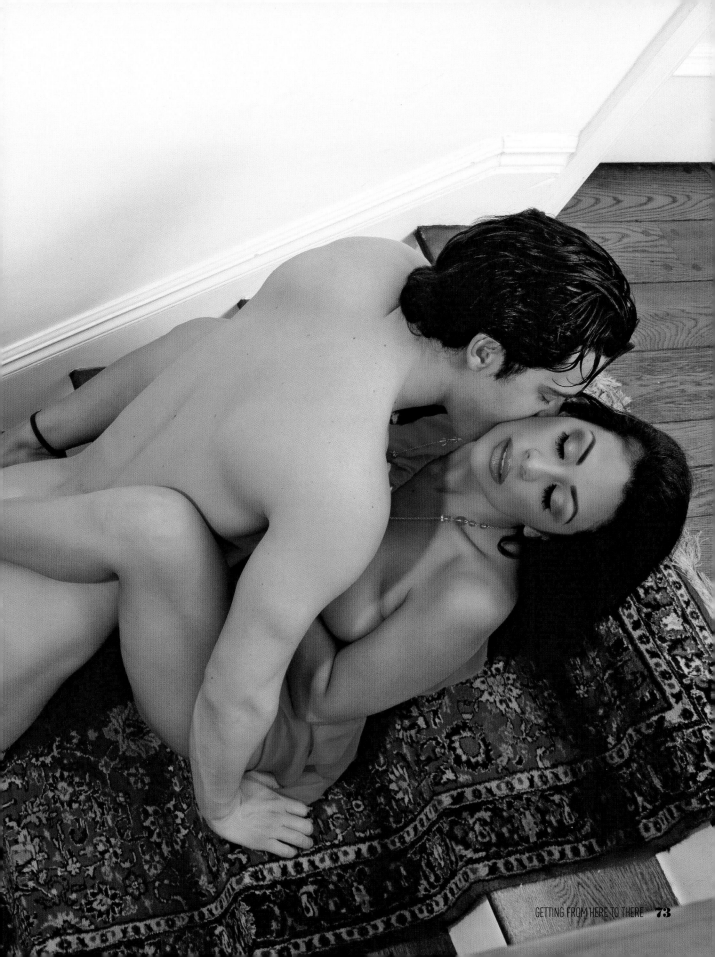

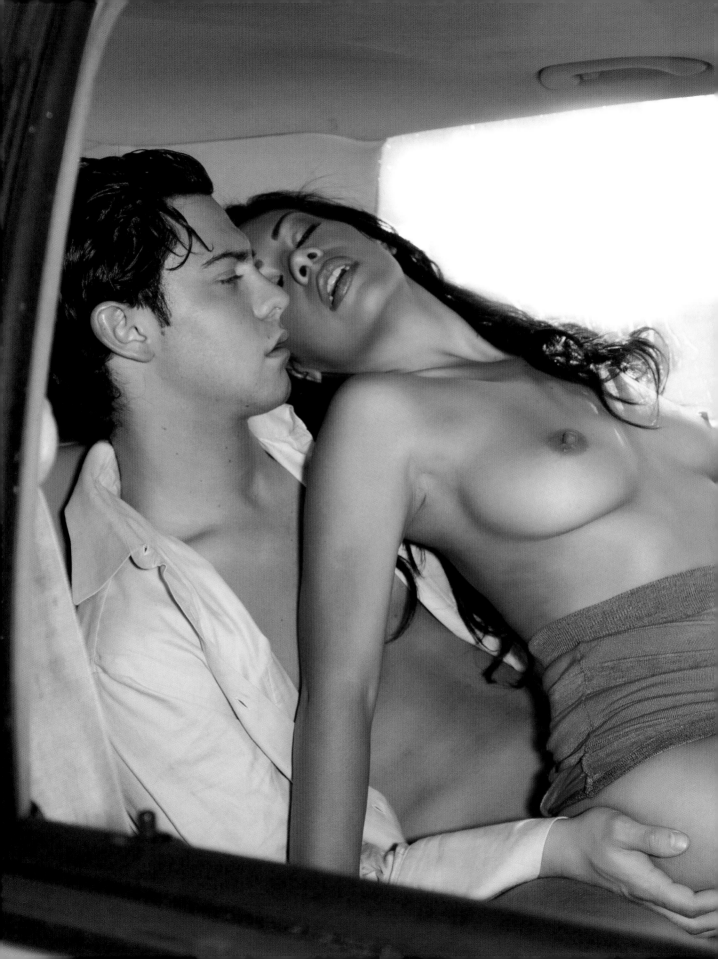

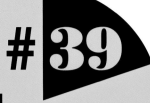

BACKSEAT SEX IN THE CAR WASH

Why not climb into the backseat while your car slides through the wet and slippery car wash? Getting the grime off your vehicle is an ordinary and often odious chore, but it needs to be done. And while you're at it, live up to the old hit tune, "Car Wash."

Estimated time: 5–7 minutes
What you'll need: a full car-wash treatment on the automatic cycle—including spray wax, undercoat, and double wash (the longer you spend going through the wash, the better chance you both have for reaching a climax); lube; an easy-access outfit

THE PLAY BY PLAY

1. Come prepared to play in the car and leave your underwear at home. For women, that means a skirt and no panties!

2. Clear everything out of the backseat before you drive through the car wash, and pull the front seats as far forward as you can to give you more room. Pull up to the wash, drop your money into the slot and …

3. … Crawl into the backseat.

4. You have plenty of choices of position here. It can be woman-on-top or man-on-top position, but I recommend the woman be on top with the guy sitting, which is more likely to bring both of you to orgasm *faster*. But get to it as soon as the car rolls along and the big brushes come down.

5. Gals, once you've lubed yourself up and positioned his penis inside you, begin to move up and down to build momentum. But just because you're the backseat driver doesn't mean you have to do all the work. Guys, you can wrap your hands around her hips and help her gyrate.

6. For a truly titillating experience, stimulate her breasts, belly, and clitoris while she rides you. This will be especially exciting with the sound of brushes caressing the car or loud soap sprays hitting the windshield.

7. And no matter what adjustments need to be made, keep this woman-on-top tip in mind: If he pops out at any point, just put him back in and resume the action. No biggie.

8. What's really spot-on about this position is that it puts the woman in control of the pace, motion, and depth of penetration, so she can get the kind of stimulation she needs to be sent over the edge.

9. Once the car starts going through the dry cycle, it's your cue to finish up quickly, pull on your clothes, and crawl back to the front seats with no one the wiser.

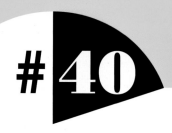

MILE-HI-JINKS

Even though sex in an airplane bathroom can be a bit of a cliché and requires ingenuity and determination, it's a trip worth taking.

Estimated time: 5–7 minutes
What you'll need: an aisle seat (nothing is worse than crawling over people, so if one of you is on the aisle, at least you can get to the bathroom with a minimum of commotion), lube, sanitary wipes

THE PLAY BY PLAY

1. You'll want to get primed for your mile-high exploit by whispering some dirty, sexy *something* while still in your seats, or throw a blanket over your laps and offer some manual stimulation as foreplay.

2. Choose a time when the bathrooms aren't busy—usually midflight. This might include meal or snack service, or right before the captain says it's okay to move about the cabin. Flight attendants are busy getting ready for service then, so it's fine to walk around.

3. Enter the bathroom separately. The first one in can clean surfaces with sanitary wipes. A few minutes later, your partner knocks gently on the door and you unlock it and let her in.

4. Since timing is crucial, this isn't an opportunity to try out new positions. The safest sex position on planes is with one partner sitting on the closed toilet seat. Lube her up generously, and your lady can slide down on you, straddling your hips. In this position, even if there's turbulence, neither of you will risk a concussion by being too close to the ceiling. If you do encounter turbulence, brace yourselves against the toilet; don't try to stand up or move.

5. A sexier position is upright wheelbarrow with your lover facing the wall, but it's not as safe.

6. Another reason to make it quick and quiet is that other people may be waiting to use the lavatory. If they're standing outside and hear sexy sounds, it may give them some suspicion about what you're doing in there—and they could call an attendant.

7. After you've reached climax, there's no time for cuddling. Pull yourselves together and exit the bathroom, but do it in a subtle way. If someone sees you leaving together, just say that one of you (decide who ahead of time) was feeling airsick and the other was there for comfort.

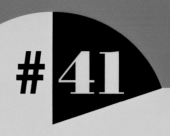

FLIGHT DELAY—HOORAY!

Stuck at the airport and already had your coffee? Well, if your flight isn't leaving for another hour and you've already checked in, explore the airport until you find a deserted hallway or stairwell. The secret is to be sure you're alone with only the *threat* of discovery. Security is testy.

Estimated time: 5 minutes or less
What you'll need: keen hearing in case someone is walking toward you

THE PLAY BY PLAY

1. After you've discovered the right hiding place, hike up your skirt or slide down your jeans, then face your guy and lean against the wall with your legs spread.

2. Next, guide his hands to the backs of your thighs and wrap your arms around his neck as he lifts you up and holds your legs snugly against his hips.

3. Plant both of your feet against the opposite wall for leverage. Or if the hallway isn't narrow enough, wrap one leg around him and plant the other foot on a piece of luggage to support your weight and give you the height to reach his pelvis.

4. This primal position is perfect for fast sex because you achieve intense clitoral contact as he presses against you to maintain the position. Plus, he gets to thrust deeply.

5. As an added bonus for him, clamp your thighs as snugly as possible around his waist. Tightening your grip will narrow the vaginal canal and create very pleasurable friction.

6. The torso-to-torso intimacy of this move means you can dive in for wet kisses to feel more connected. But try to keep one eye open just in case a security guard is making the rounds!

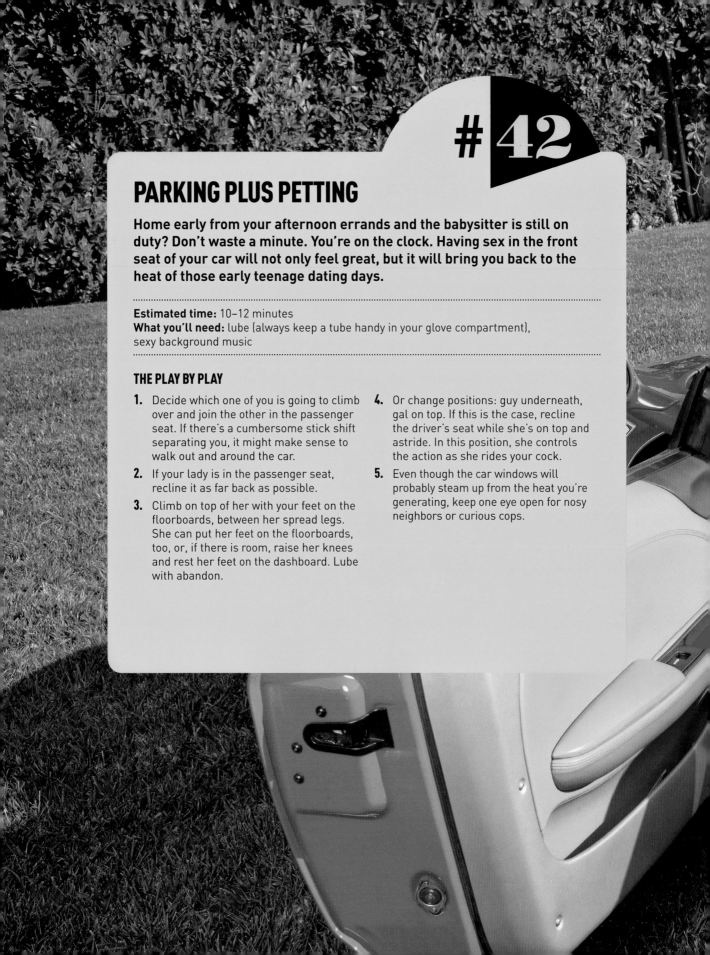

42

PARKING PLUS PETTING

Home early from your afternoon errands and the babysitter is still on duty? Don't waste a minute. You're on the clock. Having sex in the front seat of your car will not only feel great, but it will bring you back to the heat of those early teenage dating days.

Estimated time: 10–12 minutes
What you'll need: lube (always keep a tube handy in your glove compartment), sexy background music

THE PLAY BY PLAY

1. Decide which one of you is going to climb over and join the other in the passenger seat. If there's a cumbersome stick shift separating you, it might make sense to walk out and around the car.

2. If your lady is in the passenger seat, recline it as far back as possible.

3. Climb on top of her with your feet on the floorboards, between her spread legs. She can put her feet on the floorboards, too, or, if there is room, raise her knees and rest her feet on the dashboard. Lube with abandon.

4. Or change positions: guy underneath, gal on top. If this is the case, recline the driver's seat while she's on top and astride. In this position, she controls the action as she rides your cock.

5. Even though the car windows will probably steam up from the heat you're generating, keep one eye open for nosy neighbors or curious cops.

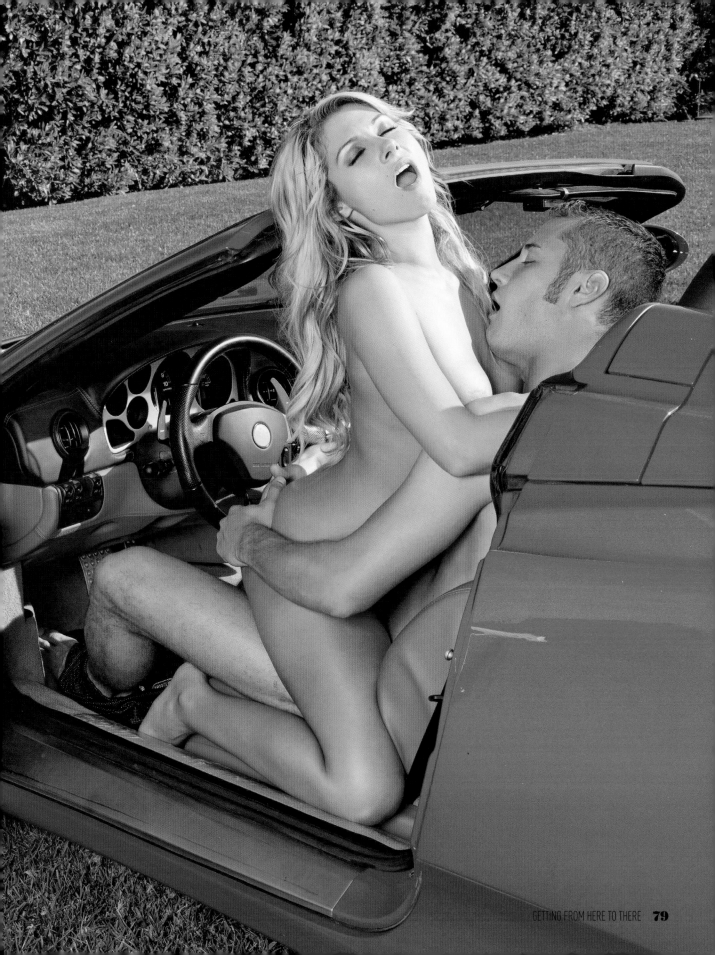

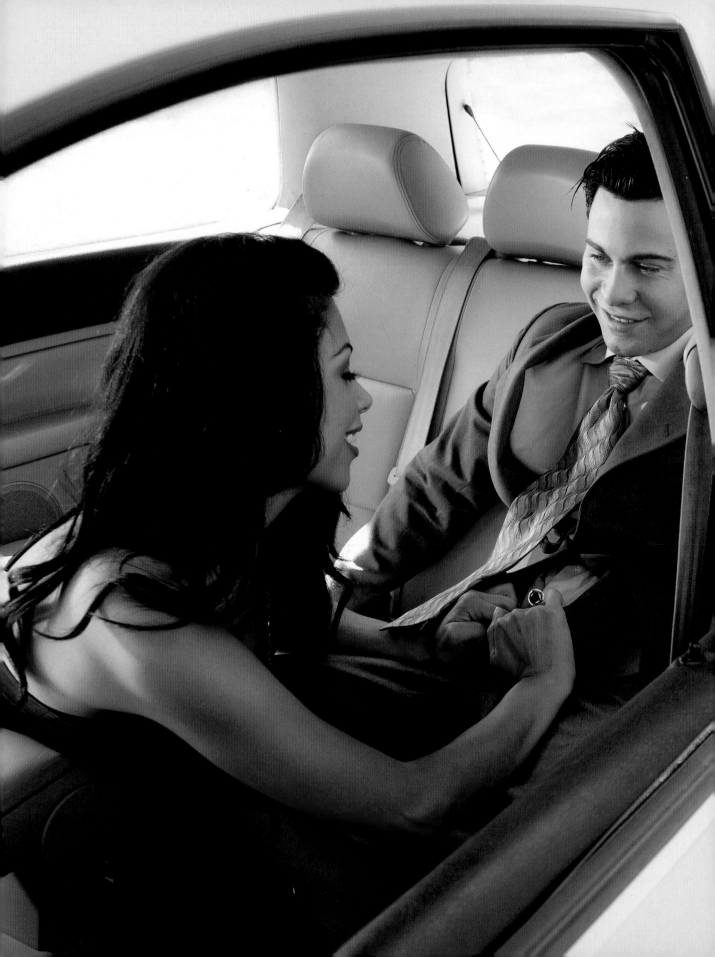

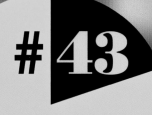

 # 43

METER-RUNNING BJ

Is sex in the back of a taxi or a luxury car a cliché? Yes! Does it feel good? Yes! You're paying for the ride and on your way. Here's how to get going.

Estimated time: 5 minutes (make sure your ride is at least that long)
What you'll need: a destination, acting skills

THE PLAY BY PLAY

1. You're on the clock, so almost immediately upon entering the cab, reach over and start rubbing your guy's crotch through his pants. He'll probably get hard by the time the meter goes up another dollar.

2. Next, unzip his fly before the next dollar appears on the meter. Then say, "Oops, I think I dropped ... my ... keys."

3. Lean over and pretend to look for your keys on the floor of the taxi, but of course go down on him with your most earnest BJ.

4. Don't forget: You can do more wonderful stuff with your mouth than just suck (and remember, the harder you suck doesn't necessarily mean the better it feels). Mix it up by licking the sensitive underside of his shaft and the nerve-ending-loaded head. Blow softly on the moistened areas; the combination of sensations will feel incredible and hopefully make him come before you reach your destination.

5. Once he's climaxed, exclaim, "Oh, here are my keys!" Lift your head and straighten your clothing.

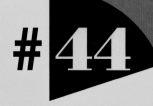

DRIVE-THRU TAFFY PULL

On a slow and boring wait at the drive-thru, before ordering your burgers and fries, burn off some pre–fast food calories by giving your honey a one-handed wank job.

Estimated time: 5 minutes or less (depending on how quickly the cars move)—and note that you can do this in two parts: pre- and postorder
What you'll need: either your spit or lube, tissues or napkins, a busy drive-thru restaurant

THE PLAY BY PLAY

1. Ladies, you're in the driver's seat with this move in more ways than one. Before you get to the ordering microphone, begin your one-handed massage by starting at the base of his penis (the part that is closest to his body) and wrapping your entire hand around it.

2. Move your lubricated hand slowly up the entire shaft and then back down again. Apply increased pressure and squeezes as he becomes more aroused.

3. After doing the up-and-down motion several times, start focusing only on the head of his cock. The head (or the glans, if you want to get all technical) is the most sensitive part of a guy's genitals, so for this area you will only need your fingers, not your entire hand. If the car needs to inch along in line, take it slowly. You don't want to rear-end the customer in front of you.

4. Now, rub the head between your thumb and index finger, alternating levels of pressure. You can also use all of your fingers and lightly massage the entire tip of the penis.

5. If he hasn't come yet and you're pulling up at the mic, throw a jacket over his lap. Continue to give him a one-handed job while you place your order.

6. Now you can pick up your meal as long as the jacket is still on his lap. Then pull into the parking area and finish the job. Keep a tissue or napkins handy.

7. Now that's what we call a *happy* meal.

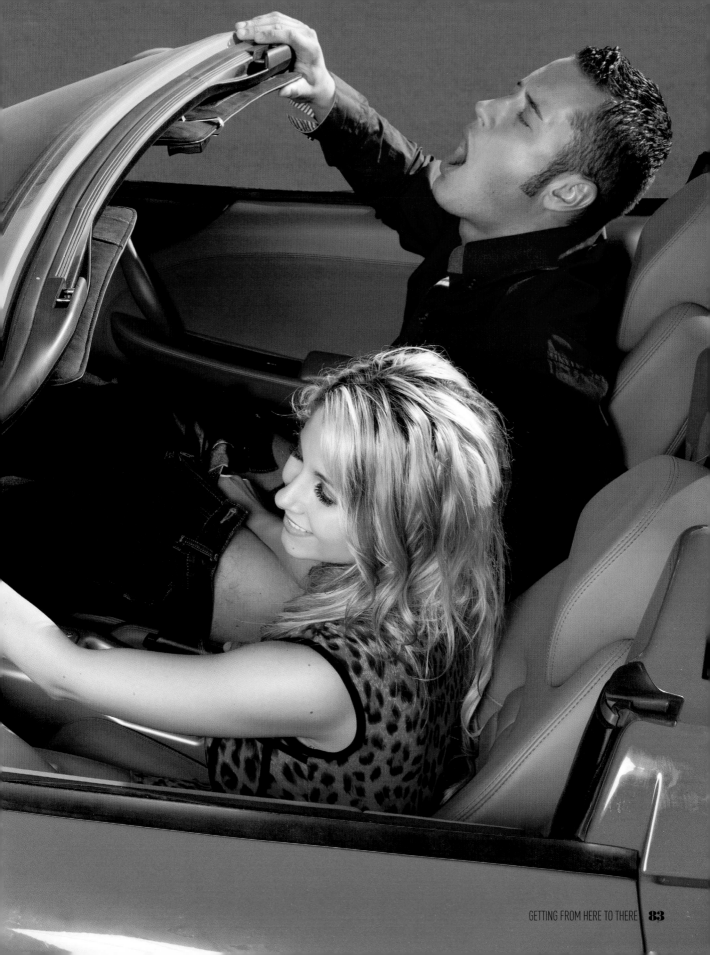

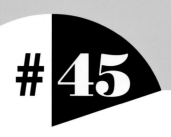

THE ROUGH RIDE HOME

If you're taking the train home after a night on the town (ladies, wear a skirt out if you can!), you're in the perfect place to get on track for memorable sex. Try these creative ways to disguise your daring and dirty deed. Obviously, keep one eye open for roving transit cops or overly observant riders.

Estimated time: 5 minutes
What you'll need: an empty train car, skirt on your lady, courage, a backpack

THE PLAY BY PLAY

1. Ladies, feeling sexy? Lean against the subway pole and assume a sexy pose.

2. Guys, here's your cue. Slip your back-pack off and onto her shoulders, so the bag is covering her front, not back (backwards, essentially).

3. Sit down and tug the straps lightly so she falls back onto your lap, facing away from you. This not only binds her to you with the thrill of your dominating force, but also helps keep things a bit more hidden; feel free to move the bag around as needed to cover any fleshy exposures.

4. Thanks to the backpack and her on your lap, no one else can see the bulge in your pants. Relax for a moment as your bodies sway to the rhythm and vibrations of the train as it moves along the track.

5. Once you feel her heating up, hike her skirt up a bit and place your middle finger in your mouth to moisten it. Reach under and go in and out of her in high speed.

6. Make sure you're positioned securely so that you can keep your steady and ensure that your finger is going in at full capacity.

7. Your goal is to get her to reach orgasm before the next stop. If she's seems distracted by the possibility to getting caught, pinch her behind with your other hand to focus her attention.

8. If the train truly is completely empty and you feel like the risk is worth it, take out your cock and give her the best train ride of her life.

FERRIS WHEEL FRICTION

While the kids are off with their friends at the amusement park, go on your own sky-high adventure. The surge of adrenaline and endorphins while you're flying down the roller coaster, going through the pitch-black haunted house, or circling on the Ferris wheel will intensify your orgasms to a thrilling degree.

Estimated time: 3–6 minutes (depending on ride time)
What you'll need: the backseat, a roomy jacket or sweater, a book of ride tickets

THE PLAY BY PLAY

1. First of all, don't forget that safety comes first. Even the seemingly tame Ferris wheel can tip dangerously if you're doing the down and dirty, so always stay buckled in.

2. One of the most exciting and easiest ways to get off when you're in public is the tried-and-true hand job. On an amusement park ride, it's even more thrilling because your adrenaline is surging super high.

3. Even though you think no one can see you, put a jacket or sweater over your laps to cover your erotic bases.

4. Guys, lick your fingers and slide them into her excited pussy. Gals, take out his works and let them feel the air before starting to fondle and pump. A word of caution to both: be careful that a fright doesn't translate into sudden jerky movements. Keep calm and steady.

5. If you're feeling daring, when you're at the top of the Ferris wheel, and both into the "ride," use your free hand wave to the crowd below. They'll have no idea how bad you're really being and your endorphins will surge even higher.

6. The good news is you don't need to worry about stifling moans and screams. Everybody else is doing it, just for a slightly different reason.

7. If the ride is too short to achieve orgasm, go for another ride, or move onto the next. You might consider investing in a book of tickets and building up momentum one ride after the next.

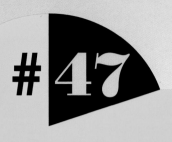

 # 47

FERRY FROLICK

Ahoy, mate! If you're going from point A to point B on a ferry, the wind and surf will certainly kick up erotic enthusiasm. The key is for women to forgo panties and wear a dress. So, ladies, feel the sea breeze—and hopefully something else!

Estimated time: 3–8 minutes
What you'll need: a steady seat, the ability to maintain your sea legs, a skirt (without panties underneath), a large blanket

THE PLAY BY PLAY

1. Matey, sit on your captain's lap, but face away from him and stare out at the bright blue sparkling sea. Let the waves move you rhythmically.

2. Pull up your skirt, and let your bare ass continue to move up and down. This should make your man's shaft nice and hard. Keep a blanket handy in case you're worried about onlookers.

3. Guys, when the time is right, pull out your eager cock and guide it inside your lady. If she's a little dry, lick your fingers and insert them first to get her juices flowing.

4. While she's still feeling filled and swaying to the rhythm of the seas, add your own jiggle and thump. Lift her up and down to increase the pressure on her clit and your cock.

5. If anyone walks by, grab that blanket! To the other ferry-goers, it will look as though your lady is innocently sitting on your lap and enjoying the waves and view. The combination of clandestine sexual activity and sea breezes can make this a Titanic-size encounter, minus the catastrophe.

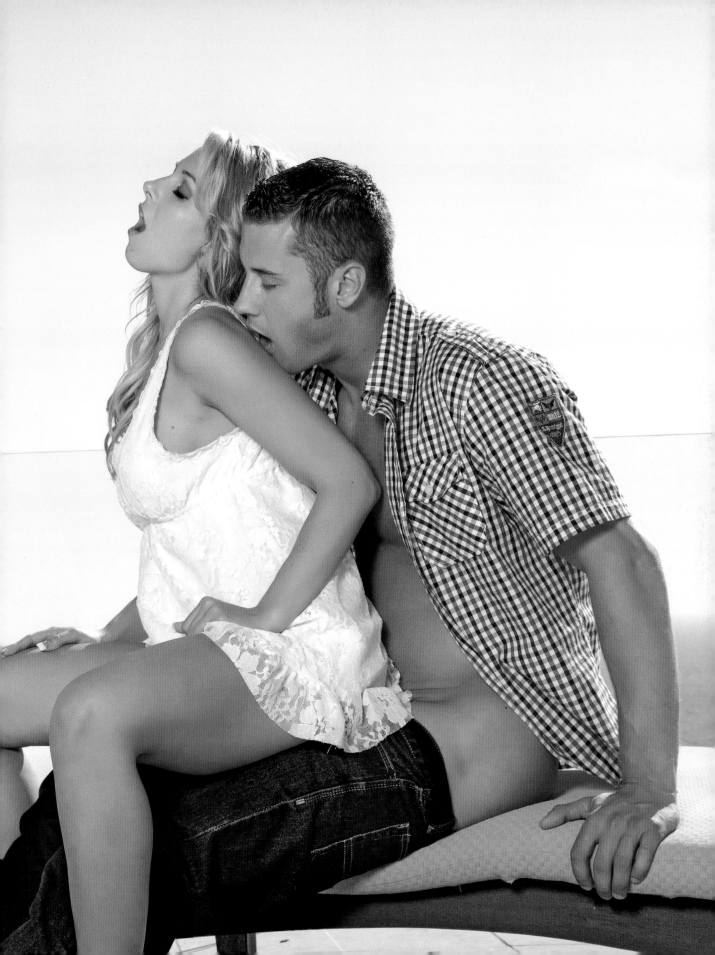

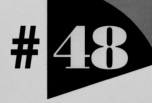

TRAFFIC JAM RELEASE

When you're at a halt in traffic and wasting precious time, lots of frustration builds up. Why not let it loose? One-third of motorists say they fantasize about sex while stuck in traffic, anyway. And 11 percent of men admit to masturbating while driving. So take the pressure off the horn and put it between your own legs.

Estimated time: 5–7 minutes
What you'll need: lube (keep it handy in the glove compartment), tissues, jacket or light blanket

THE PLAY BY PLAY

1. If you want to be in control of what, when, and who gets a peek at your gutsy exhibition, before you unzip/ pull your pants down/ lift your skirt/push your panties to the side, place jackets or a light blanket over your laps.

2. You've probably been masturbating for years now, so you know what works quickly to get you to climax. Doing it in the car with the possibility of being watched heightens arousal and speeds up the action. (Keep in mind that truckers really do have a bird's eye view, though.) If you still want to up the ante, roll down the windows—or even better, flash your boobs to passing motorists.

3. Meanwhile, feel free to reach across and touch your partner while you're pleasuring yourself. But gals, if he's stroking his penis and has a rhythm going, don't stroke his rod now. Be open to caressing and fondling any other part of his body instead—thighs, stomach, arms, and nipples. Guys, vice versa.

4. While one of you is masturbating, the other can just watch also. This is both arousing and informative. If you choose this technique, your partner's orgasm is your cue to begin pleasuring yourself.

5. You can also attempt to reach synchronized orgasms. Harmonize by talking dirty to each other and describing how close you are to coming. If you're concerned about fellow motorists hearing you, turn the music up. If you're not, whoop, holler, and moan loudly.

6. As sexual tension rises, keep going, even if you're nervous about traffic starting or stopping again at any moment. Allow the pleasant feeling to win over and you'll be increasingly excited and won't want to stop. When that happens, you'll reach the ultimate climax.

7. Your choice on whether you want to honk or not.

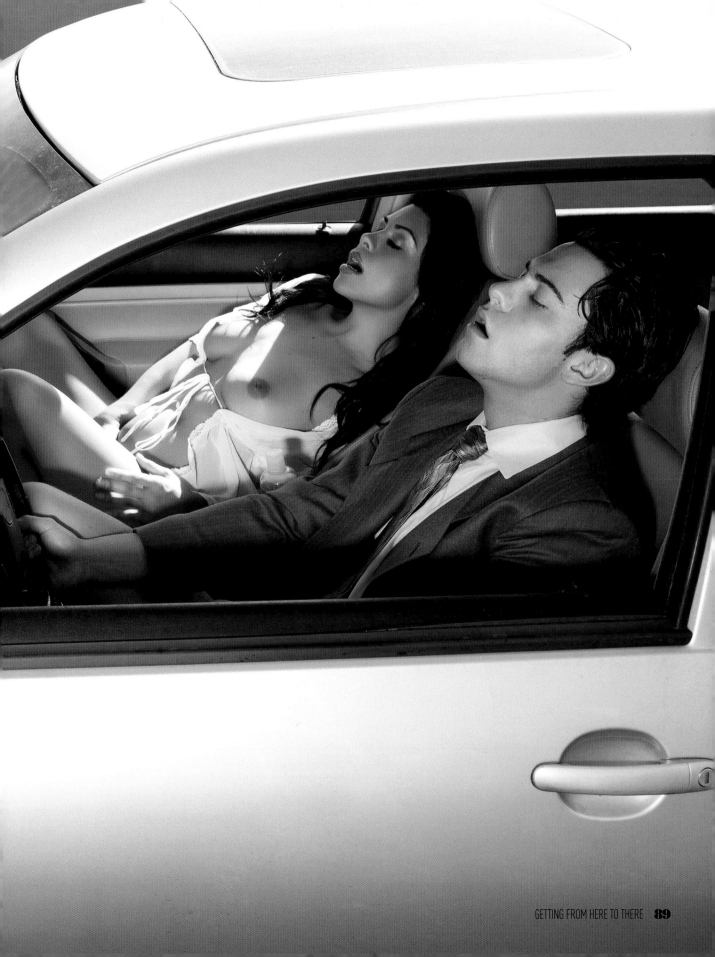

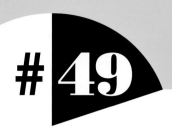

REVVING UP

Whether the garage is attached to your home or under your apartment or house, there's something sexy about the gritty, dank feel of it. You're there to get your automobile, but before you take off, get things going on the hood of your car.

Estimated time: 6–10 minutes
What you'll need: a garage or out-of-the-way place to park the car, a car radio/ CD /iPod, an automobile

THE PLAY BY PLAY

1. If you're parked in a public garage, you might want to first drive your car to a more secluded area where other customers won't be wandering (try the top level).

2. You know you're going to be going at it, but you don't have all the time in the world. Turn the music on and give yourselves two to three songs to climax. Something with a hard and pounding beat is best.

3. Without further discussion, lift your lover's skirt or pull down her pants and place her bare bottom on the bonnet of the car. Your rough handling and the cool feel of the metal will be a shocking turn-on for your lady, especially if she's used to a more tender touch.

4. As long as you're both in the mood, you can continue to role-play as the gruff lover. Keep one ear on the background music in case you have to exert even more desperate pressure as time runs out.

5. Without uttering a word, change to oral. Spread her legs wide and then lift them onto your shoulders. This is known as the headlock position. Start off licking her in slow motion and then pick up speed as if you were a driving force to be reckoned with. Keep going until she reaches her destination—or the songs come to an end.

6. Hopefully your lover has been satisfied in time. If there's still some time left or you want to start the two- or three-song game over again, demand she return the attention and switch positions; this time you sit on the car hood while she leans over and sucks you off.

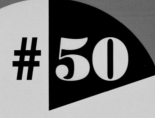

#50

DRIVE-IN FLICK TO REMEMBER

Thank goodness it's movie night and the babysitter is on duty. This time rather than opting for the regular cinema, consider a drive-in movie. It might just be the hottest ticket in town.

Estimated time: 12 minutes, or as long as you want
What you'll need: a comfortable car, a drive-in movie theater, lube

THE PLAY BY PLAY

1. Tonight promises to bring you back to your early days of dating, when just feeling up your date could get you going. Be prepared to steam up the car windows!

2. Once you've pulled into your parking spot, turn down the movie's sound track because it can be distracting and break the mood. You can always turn on your own music if you like.

3. The great thing about screwing in a car is that you have options depending on which "route" you want to take. And regardless of which you choose, they'll all garner 5-star reviews.

4. Option 1: This works best if you're both thin and flexible. Guys, sitting in the driver's seat, push the seat back as far as it can go. If you have a tilt steering wheel, tilt it back too. Then, have your star straddle you in the seat. Sit up slightly and thrust into her using the steering wheel to pull yourself forward.

5. Option 2: Put the seats down and have her kneel one knee on the back of each seat (right on the driver's side, left on the passenger's). Her hands should be on the backseat or backseat floor holding her up. Carefully get behind (also kneeling) and ride her doggie style (being ever so careful not to bump your head).

6. Option 3: Another choice? You might consider opting for what is probably the most comfortable of all auto sex positions. Push the front seats as far forward as you can and lie down in the back seat while she rides you. As Jude Law said in the movie *Alfie*, "This was President Kennedy's favorite position."

7. For a romantic ending to your personal flick of the week, cuddle close as you get caught up on the plot.

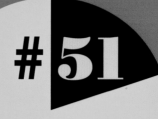

ELEVATOR INTERCOURSE

You're both on your way somewhere—maybe to see the accountant, to dinner at a rooftop restaurant, to a friend's apartment. You might as well enjoy getting there. Elevators are a perfect place to have very hot and fast sex.

Estimated time: 3–5 minutes
What you'll need: a sense of adventure, a certain amount of flexibility

THE PLAY BY PLAY

1. Riding several floors won't be enough time to get either of you off, so you'll need to be brave and stall the elevator. Be careful not to trigger any alarms—you don't want the fire department coming to your rescue!

2. Look for a camera. If you find one, stand right beneath it so it only has a partial view. It's even better if you can position yourselves completely out of the way. In any case, try to avoid being identified.

3. When it comes to elevator sex, time is crucial (unless you enjoy getting caught). It's best if you each undo your own clothing. Since time is of the essence, it's not necessary to remove all your clothes.

4. The best position for this kind of fast encounter is known as standing spoons. Gals, turn around so your back is to your man and you're facing the elevator wall.

5. Guys, embrace your woman with one arm and use the other to position yourself. You can also use your free hand to help guide your penis into her pussy.

6. You'll both need to bend your knees slightly like two spoons pressing together. Try to move in unison, pushing and pumping and keeping the penetration deep and intense.

7. Because the entry was made from the rear, there's an excellent chance your lady's G-spot and clitoris will be stimulated, offering optimum opportunity for each partner to climax.

8. Once you're done, be sure to button, zip, and generally tidy your appearance.

9. Let the elevator run again, but it's a good idea if you don't exit on the floor of your destination. Stop the elevator one flight before and walk up the stairs.

LOCATION! LOCATION! LOCATION!
Taking It Out of Bounds for Increased Excitement

Sex in public is a favorite sexual fantasy. The possibility of getting caught or being watched can be a steamy turn-on for lots of couples. Getting down and dirty while taking it out from behind the safety of locked doors, and possibly out in the public eye, often satisfies the desire to crank up the risk factor.

The boost that accompanies a fast public encounter actually initiates a real physical reaction in our bodies. It's known as the "fight or flight response" because a cocktail of stress-related hormones (adrenaline, noradrenaline, and cortisol) is released into our bloodstream, which makes our heart rate increase and blood rush to our head and muscles. When this happens, our primal animal selves are geared up to either fight or escape in a hurry as if it's a matter of life or death. The thrill often brings on a quicker and more intense orgasm.

Whether it's in a restaurant's bathroom, a park or beach, a movie theater or the supermarket, this chapter gives you the PLAY BY PLAY so your next public appearance lands you a triple-X rating.

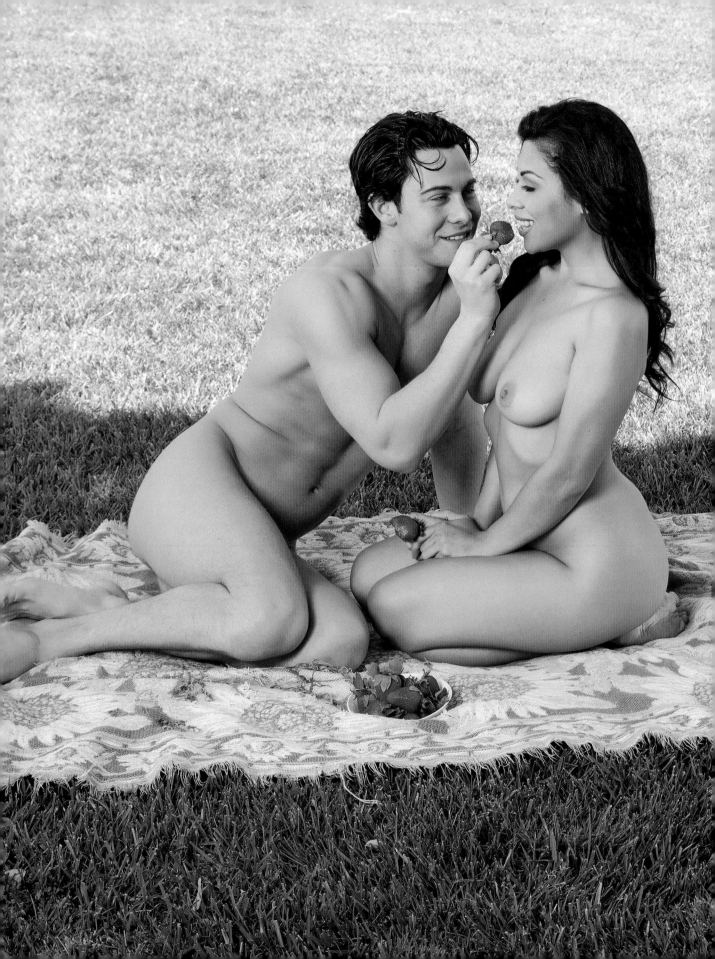

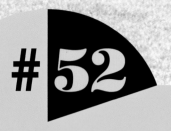

PICK YOUR OWN PRODUCE

If you like to get your hands dirty, check out an orchard or a farm and pick your own apples, peaches, or berries—whatever is in season. You'll find plenty of places begging for sweet action. As an added perk, you can make a dessert or jam afterward with your "hard"-earned ingredients.

Estimated time: 5 minutes
What you'll need: a blanket

THE PLAY BY PLAY

1. Begin tantalizing each other by feeding your lover just-picked juicy fruits.

2. Now lie down on the blanket where there are no roots or rocks and fall to the ground like a horny Adam and Eve in your own Garden of Eden.

3. Eve, since you're the seductress, move yourself on top of Adam so that your clit is right in front of his fruit-drenched lips.

4. Your mouth, meanwhile, hovers above his cock.

5. Enjoy this forbidden, fresh-air version of 69, but take care not to strain your necks. Because you're giving and receiving pleasure at the same time, some claim 69 is the ultimate erotic sensation. Others find it to be ultimately *frustrating*: It's all too easy to get lazy on your end. If your partner's working his magic and you're about to climax, it's common to forget about his pleasure and try to get away with a few lackluster licks. Big mistake, ladies: 69 is a great way to add naughtiness and variety.

6. Because a 69 exposes the entire pelvic region, giving him access to the whole of your vulva, perineum (the hairless bit between the anus and the vaginal opening), and anus, he's able to stimulate much more than just your clitoris. In fact, some men consider 69 so erotic, they ejaculate too quickly—literally two licks in. This is why it's advisable for him to start working on you long before you start on him.

7. If your guy is slower to react and it's too awkward and tiring to attempt to use only your mouth to stimulate him, use your hands as well. And don't be scared to remove your mouth and work on him with your hands to give yourself a break. Ditto for the guys.

8. Note: Avoid conversations with snakes in the grass.

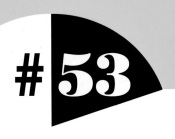

COMING-ATTRACTION SEX

Okay, you *finally* found time to see a movie in a real theater! You're even early, but neither of you is interested in watching endless, over-the-top trailers. Here is your chance to take entertainment into your own hands before the main feature begins. You'll want to choose a movie that's not too popular, and one that's playing in a newer theater where the armrests fold up.

Estimated time: 8–12 minutes
What you'll need: jackets, lube, a fairly empty movie theater, soda and popcorn

THE PLAY BY PLAY

1. Buy popcorn and a large drink with plenty of ice and bring it to your seats. Slide up the armrest that's between you. Guys, place the drink firmly in the armrest's cup holder on your other side.

2. Place your jackets over your laps and begin to pleasure each other simultaneously. Gals, take out the lube from your purse and gently rub some on his penis. Move your fist up and down on his shaft in a slow and steady motion.

3. Variety is the key, so mix up your speed and pressure as his arousal grows.

4. Guys, while you're getting off, don't forget to take care of your lady. Since she's probably not adequately self-lubricated, squeeze some lube on your fingers, and then use the tips of your index and middle fingers to rub her clitoris softly in a circular motion.

5. Continue your pace but add a thrilling coming attraction of your own: Reach into the soda cup with your other hand and grab one or two ice cubes. Tell her to stay still so you don't disturb your fellow movie-goers.

6. Now rub the ice along your lover's inner thighs, from her knees to her mound. Roll it around her pubic hair while you begin to increase the speed of clitoris rubbing with your other hand. If she gasps out loud, tell her put some popcorn in her mouth to muffle the noise.

7. If she whispers, "Don't stop!" then don't stop. Some women, however, like it when you take a break from the clitoris and proceed to insert those very same fingers inside the vagina at a rhythmic pace. If that's her choice, first slip the ice along her pussy lips. Careful not to insert all the way.

8. Ladies, keep working your right-hand magic. Your guy may need to keep that soda straw in his mouth to cover up his own happy breathing.

9. Try to synchronize your finales a few minutes before the main feature begins so you have time to clean up before the real show begins.

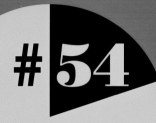

GROCERY SHOPPING WITH GOOD VIBRATIONS

All those cucumbers, bananas, and carrots—it's no wonder we get horny at the supermarket. Guys can take advantage of the natural turn-on by secretly controlling your hidden remote-controlled vibrator while you're looking for ripe produce or scanning the cereal aisle. Grocery shopping has never been so climactic.

Estimated time: 12 minutes or less
What you'll need: a portable, remote-controlled vibrator with a range of at least 25 feet (7.5m); the ability to stifle cries of ecstasy; a shopping list

THE PLAY BY PLAY

1. Test the remote-controlled vibrator at home to ensure the batteries are working and to prepare in advance for your reaction. You might not want to be screaming out "Oh, oh, oh, OH!" at the supermarket. Besides, one of the most exciting aspects of a remote vibrator is the fact that while your sexual excitement is mounting, those around you have no idea.

2. Ladies, put the vibrator in your panties, and guys, grab that remote. Now head to the store.

3. Guys, understand you now have total control over your lady's clit. Be both sneaky and sensitive. While she's fondling a banana for ripeness or checking the price of strawberry preserves, zap the remote. The surprise factor is a huge turn-on. Keep her on edge by setting the vibrator off at irregular intervals, trying to pick the moments when you'll get her the most excited. For example, you might zap her just as she's asking a clerk where she can find the avocados or while she's weighing the grapes or pushing the cart down a narrow aisle.

4. If your lover reacts openly with little or loud squeals, sternly remind her she'll have to remain calm and unruffled or you won't give her any more thrills. Remember: You are in charge. *Totally.*

5. Get your own charge as you watch while her knees buckle or she whimpers quietly. Try to draw out the excitement and anticipation. By the time she has filled the grocery cart, your lady should barely be able to walk a steady line.

6. She's primed to the max. As soon as you reach the car, finger her and she'll have several orgasms in a matter of seconds.

7. One cautionary note: Remote-controlled vibrators are quiet, but they *are* vibrators. Don't think you'll get away with your little game if the supermarket is quiet. Hope for the volume of mind-numbing Muzak to be turned up loud.

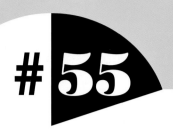

 # 55

SEX IN THE STACKS

A recent survey shows that in order to save money, there's been an uptick in the number of people borrowing books from their local library rather than buying them. If you're joining these thrifty bookworms, take advantage of the library's quiet policy to have hush-hush sex.

Estimated time: 3–5 minutes
What you'll need: a library during nonpeak hours, restraint, clothing that's easy to take off or lift up, a bookwormish attitude

THE PLAY BY PLAY

1. Having sex in a library is all about planning. Scope the place out first, and find some of the more secluded and quiet sections of the building.

2. Sex in the corridors, between shelves and books, means the tight spaces will give you and your partner the opportunity to explore new sexual positions—mostly standing ones. These positions also allow for easy retreat in the case of possible discovery.

3. What you wear is important. Guys should remember to wear pants with a zipper, and boxer shorts rather than briefs for easier access. Women should wear skirts with no underwear rather than pants.

4. Great library sex means a fast orgasm. Guys, lean against a sturdy shelf while standing erect in front of your lady.

5. Remain strong while she wraps her legs more or less around your waist. Now unzip your pants and pull out your cock. You might want to finger her for a few minutes to get her wet.

6. Now slide deeply into her vagina. If she yelps with pleasure, a quiet "shh" will remind your lovely where you are before a librarian makes an appearance. Remember that sound travels in large spaces.

7. While holding her buttocks, draw her pelvis toward you. This position allows you to face each other and silently exchange caresses while you move slowly in and out until you climax, hopefully along with your studious partner.

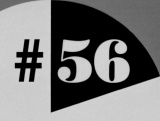

BLEACHER FINGERBAITING

The adrenaline release and roars of the big sports-loving crowd will help get you both heated up. Of course, you may not want to miss a crucial play since you've paid big bucks for the event, but if it's a yawner or during halftime, squeeze in a play of your own.

Estimated time: 5 minutes or less
What you'll need: a roomy blanket or big jacket, poker faces, trust in the gods of good sportsmanship (that you won't miss an important play)

THE PLAY BY PLAY

1. As soon as halftime begins, grab the blankets or your jackets and pull your lady onto your lap facing the field. If you get any strange looks, just shrug them off and give your gal a winning hug.

2. Throw the blanket or jackets over both of you so her bottom is completely covered and you feel cozy and protected.

3. Now slip both your hands beneath the blanket and spread her legs apart, lifting her skirt or unzipping her jeans. By this time, there's a good chance no one is paying much attention since there's a halftime show going on.

4. Just let your hands rest there on her mound for a minute or two. Tease her with no action and let her taste the excruciating thrill of wanting more.

5. When the crowd cheers with appreciation and you think she just can't stand it anymore, put your first two fingers together and place them over the top of her clitoris. Rub her in slow, sexy circles. Vary your speed and pressure (but not too hard) until you find something that drives her wild. You'll know because she'll be squirming in the most delightful way.

6. Many women masturbate exactly like this, so don't be surprised if her body responds and she comes quickly. If that's the case, whisper in her ear "More?" If her reply is yes, then guide her hands and place them between her legs on top of her pubes. Even if she resists, be persistent. Cup your hand over hers and coax her to pleasure herself while you add just the right amount of heat and pressure.

7. When you know she's reached her goal, help her get her clothing back on, give her butt a sporting tap, and enjoy the rest of the show.

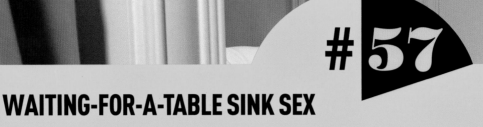

#57

WAITING-FOR-A-TABLE SINK SEX

The hostess tells you there's a half-hour wait for a table and suggests a drink at the bar. Not a bad idea, but here's a better way to spend your waiting time. Just be sure to make it quick—the goal is to get your sex fix and keep your table too!

Estimated time: 5–7 minutes
What you'll need: a single-occupancy bathroom, lube, dramatic flair

THE PLAY BY PLAY

1. Pretend nothing out of the ordinary is going to happen. Just stroll over to the bar like any loving couple and order your drinks.

2. While sipping your cocktails, make a plan to meet in the men's bathroom (where there will likely be less traffic). Guys, you go first, so excuse yourself, offer a peck on your date's cheek, and head to the bathroom.

3. A few minutes later, tell the bartender you'll be right back and follow your guy's lead. Knock on the door and whisper your name, just to be sure all is clear.

4. Guys, you should be waiting with your pants down and ready for action.

5. You don't want to waste any time. Prop your lady against the sink and help edge her elbows and butt so that they're leaning into the basin.

6. For fast public-bathroom sex, the best position is standing missionary because she can wrap her leg around you and you're facing each other. Lean against the wall or sink for support.

7. After you've made her nice and wet with lube, move inside her and thrust—but not too hard. Pressure against the sink could be painful for her. Plus, you know how tiring one-way thrusting can get.

8. Luckily, you probably won't have to maintain this position for long. Fear of being caught turns up the speed of a climax even more.

9. When you've both been reached orgasm, check your reflections in the mirror to make sure you're presentable, and then leave the bathroom separately.

10. Your drinks are waiting at the bar. Why not toast to your smoldering sexual attraction?

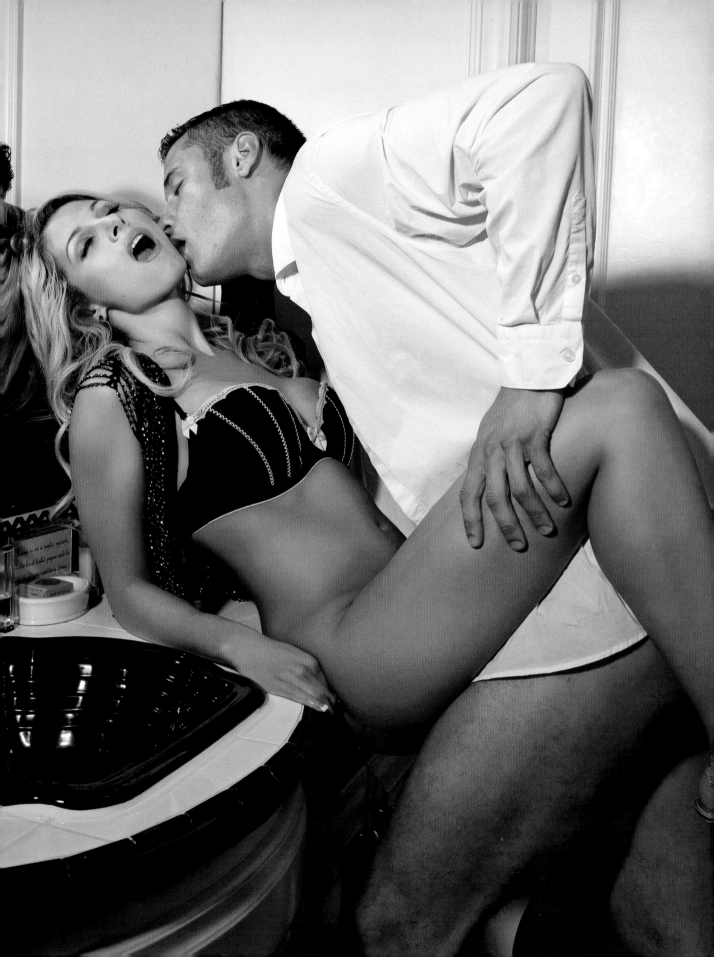

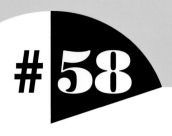

 # 58

RELATIVE O

You've both been dreading the annual visit to Aunt Tilly's and the required family get-together. The good news is that family gatherings are an excellent way to get it on with a tinge of underlying naughtiness. Who would have thought you kids could be so bad?

Estimated time: 10–12 minutes
What you'll need: lube (carry it in your pocket), a locked bathroom

THE PLAY BY PLAY

1. Get horny on the drive to the relatives' homestead by talking graphically about all the things you're going to do to each other without uptight Aunt Tilly suspecting a thing. If your kids are in the car, text or pass notes instead.

2. Once you arrive and after about an hour of niceties, confirm your arrangement to meet upstairs in the bathroom, where you're sure there will be a lock on the door.

3. Guys, tell Aunt Tilly you're headed upstairs for a quick nap or to unpack. Then get ready for action; it's always nice if you've gotten your cock hard with self-stroking before your honey shows up.

4. Ladies, while you're with Aunt Tilly, tell her you feel unkempt from traveling and would like to take a shower. Hopefully she'll oblige.

5. Guys, as soon as your partner walks through the bathroom door, take her by surprise and grab her from behind. Don't forget to lock the door and start the shower running—of course you're not taking one, but you don't want Tilly to suspect a thing. Also, be quick about it. You don't want anyone looking for you.

6. Now yank up her skirt. Apply the lube that you had in your pocket and then engage in standing rear-entry sex. She can support herself on the sink while you thrust, slowly and gently at first, and then more forcefully. The steam from the shower will increase the intensity.

7. Guys, you'll probably climax quickly, but you want to be sure that your sweetie also has an O. So, at the same you're moving in and out, rub her clit with a constant rhythm. Whisper in her ear, "Is this feeling good? Do you want me to make you come another way?" Then listen carefully to her instruction and obey until she's satisfied.

8. Make sure you're both presentable before returning to the relatives—and hide that lube tube well!

SEX IN THE SWIMMING POOL

Well, there you are—hot, slippery, *and* wet, and gazing at each other in your scanty swimsuits. But hold on! Sex in a swimming pool isn't safe unless you promise to stay in the shallow end.

Estimated time: 3–8 minutes
What you'll need: silicone lubricant, which is not water-soluble; the shallow end of a pool; an ability to relax and float; sexy bathing suits

THE PLAY BY PLAY

1. The great advantage of swimming-pool sex is that you can do it undetected, without having to strip. Gals, just push your bathing suit to the side to expose your crotch, and guys, do the same for your works. It helps if you're wearing skimpy suits because a.) your sexy attire will help turn each other on, and b.) skimpy suits make it easier to expose the good bits.

2. Now guys, stand leaning against the side of the pool and rub her vaginal area with non-water-soluble lube. When she's ready to be penetrated, do it while she floats on her back and places her feet on your chest. You can support her by holding her afloat with your hands underneath her back.

3. If this position isn't to your liking or you want to switch it around, have her straddle you with her arms around your neck and her legs floating freely at your sides.

4. Or sit on the pool stairs and let her straddle you sitting backward.

5. One word of caution: Even great swimmers shouldn't try to screw in the deep end of the pool. This puts couples at risk for awkward moments of gulping water at best, and drowning at worst.

6. As soon as you're both satisfied, pull your bathing suits back in place and leave the pool together. You might want to take warm showers to rinse off the chlorine and love juices. It's even better if you can shower together.

TIPPING IN THE COATROOM

P-a-r-t-y! Well, it's about time you guys found the time! All parties have a place to throw coats and belongings—usually in the bedroom and on the bed. How convenient! This is an ideal place for oral sex, but it does carry some risks. Obviously, someone might come in to get or leave his coat; however, odds are probably remote if it's midway through the party. This also works if you're the hosts. Hopefully, there's a lock on the door.

Estimated time: 6–10 minutes
What you'll need: your own coats, excellent timing, a handy excuse if you're asked where you were, a lock on the coatroom door (ideally)

THE PLAY BY PLAY

1. Make a plan to meet in the bedroom. Guys, get there first and prepare the area by finding your own coats and laying them on top of the others.

2. Gals, when you get in the room lift your skirt and slide your butt on top of your coats. Sit on the edge of the bed with your knees apart so your man can kneel between your legs.

3. This position is terrific for vaginal and G-spot stimulation, and it's also perfect should you have to quickly compose yourselves in case someone walks in while you're doing the dirty.

4. Okay, she's ready and primed. So guys, pull your lover forward for better access and hold her hips for support. If someone knocks on the door and yells he's got to get in to get his coat, just respond that you'll be right out—that you're having an emergency.

5. Now get busy. While sucking her clitoris slowly insert two fingers into her vagina, palm facing upward. Feel along her upper wall until you find her G-spot, and then stroke it firmly while continuing to suck her clitoris using the same rhythm until she whimpers with satisfaction.

6. This is your gift to your girl. She'll go back to the party beaming, knowing she has the best lover in the room.

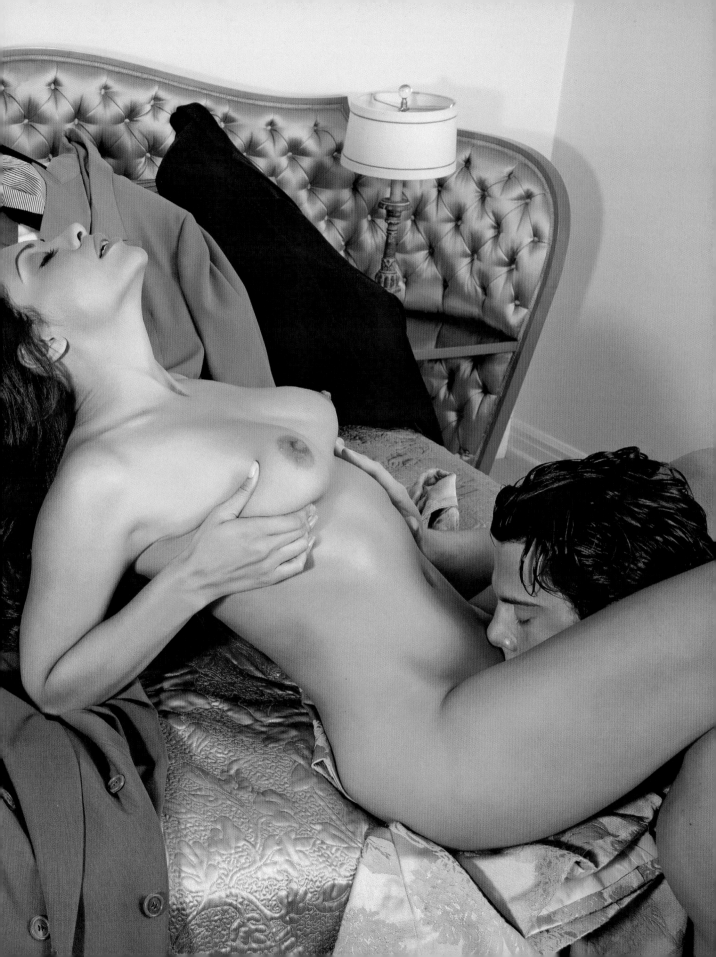

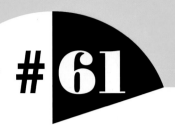

DINING OUT HORS D'OEUVRES

Let's get real. A woman can't just slide under a restaurant table and offer her man a blow job. Who are you? Samantha Jones? But if you're sitting next to each other, there's no reason why you can't slip your hands under the tablecloth and enjoy the sensations.

Estimated time: 3 minutes
What you'll need: a secluded table in the corner of a restaurant or a roomy booth

THE PLAY BY PLAY

1. Have the hostess seat you next to each other rather than across from your partner. But don't let this arrangement keep you from staring into each other's eyes. Just turn your heads and gaze with the intimate feelings you're both sharing in this moment.

2. Reach under the table, and using opposite hands, touch your partner by rubbing, stroking, and massaging. Or, if you prefer, this position also works to heighten arousal just as well if you choose to touch yourselves. Go ahead, do whatever feels good for you. None of the other diners can see a thing.

3. Either one you choose, this position allows you to continue to gaze into each other's eyes, heightening the sensation of adoration and sexual bonding. Pay attention to your partner's facial expressions of pleasure. Whatever your lover expresses with silent communication, you will feel as if an electric current here running between you.

4. When you can sense your partner is reaching the limit, join in the feeling with a quiet murmur of acknowledgement. Lean over and offer a kiss.

5. Don't worry if one of you doesn't climax. The heat generated at the table will carry through to the bedroom at home.

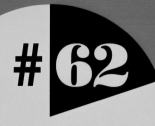

CONCERT BANGING

Practically anything goes at a rock concert, and thanks to the teeming and sweaty frenzy of a powerful beat, it can be one of the best places to get your sex drive racing.

Estimated time: 12 minutes
What you'll need: back-row seats, to keep a beat, a laissez-faire attitude

THE PLAY BY PLAY

1. When you start feeling the beat, get out of your seats and dance, dance, dance. As the intensity builds, come closer and feel free to bump and grind.

2. Don't worry—no one is looking. Guys, touch her breasts and cup her mound while she strokes your hardening shaft.

3. Once you've driven each other up the wall with desire, go to one.

4. Since you're in the last row, just walk behind the seats, but make sure there's no standing-room-only, or SRO, section.

5. With the help of the loud music and driving beat, lean your lover against the wall and force her knees apart with your legs. Then pin her hands above the wall with your free hand.

6. You can say anything you want. Feel free to swear or moan loudly. No one can hear and, frankly, no one cares.

7. Now you can sink slowly into her until you both syncopate and get a groove going. It doesn't matter how you gyrate; this is one public place where moving seductively is not only overlooked, but it's also expected. So enjoy yourselves and take it to the max.

8. If one of you climaxes first, get the groove going again until your partner also reaches the high note.

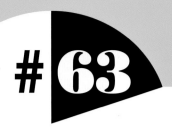

63

POOL TABLE PENETRATION

Set the balls up, and get ready to play a game of titillating billiards where you're guaranteed to bank every erotic shot. This is a game where bending the rules leads to amazingly hot plays.

Estimated time: 9–12 minutes
What you'll need: a pool table in a private area, pool cue, lube, good aim

THE PLAY BY PLAY

1. Guys, pick up your pool cue and wave it menacingly in front of your lovely opponent. Tell her to turn and bend over the table. Pull down her panties and gently tap her booty with a promise that the stakes will get higher. Make your taps harder. Perhaps harder. She'll be nice and hot for your first shot.

2. Now it's time to put your balls in play. Unzip your pants and let your works hang out rubbing against her rosy ass. Aroused?

3. While she's splayed on the table, lube up and enter her vaginally or anally with ease. Be careful not to slime up the table.

4. Ladies don't be shy. While he's inside you, insist he really take aim with his pool stick and take a shot. Call out the ball you want him to pocket. If he doesn't get it in, tell him to slip slightly out of you. Keep this game going until the ball is pocketed and he can enter fully. Simultaneous distraction and focus is guaranteed to drive you both wild.

5. If you prefer to go for another round, pool tables are extraordinarily comfy for intercourse. And you don't need to keep score.

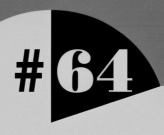

ALLEY OOPS

It's another ho-hum Tuesday night and you're feeling bored. Ask you partner to come for a walk with you to get some fresh air. While you're walking, look for dark alley or hidden nook where you can do a little role-playing. Even if you're caught, it's no big deal because people expect to see shadowy goings-on in an alley. Don't disappoint!

Estimated time: 7–10 minutes
What you'll need: clothing that exposes flesh in a flash; a dark, out-of-the-way alley; an appreciation for sordid danger; a wad of bills

THE PLAY BY PLAY

1. Sex in alleys is notorious for playing into our deepest and often darkest fantasies. If you're both game, up the ante by role-playing client and prostitute.

2. Guys, lean up against the wall and forcefully pull her close to you for a deep kiss.

3. Girls, remember you're his prostitute. This guy has nerve trying to get something for nothing! Don't go any further without demanding payment. Say huskily, "That's $100 for ten minutes!" If he balks, demand he empty his wallet, count the cash out loud, and shove it down your bra.

4. Once an agreement is reached, lean into him and let him know he can do whatever he wants to you. After all, he's paying for it.

5. Guys, go for it. Hike up her skirt, and not particularly gingerly. Remain standing and lift her leg, guiding it to hook around your waist. Unzip your pants hastily. Time is money! Then push her panties aside, push your cock inside of her and hold on to her ass while you pump.

6. Talk dirty. Tell her she's your "slut for the night" or the "hottest hooker you've ever had." Say, "Baby, you're a very bad girl and I'm going to punish you."

7. You've heard it all, Lady of the Night, so be tough. Count the minutes left. "You've got three minutes, buddy." If he doesn't reach climax in time, it's up to your heart of gold to decide whether you'll give him any "free" time—or a new way to make it up to you.

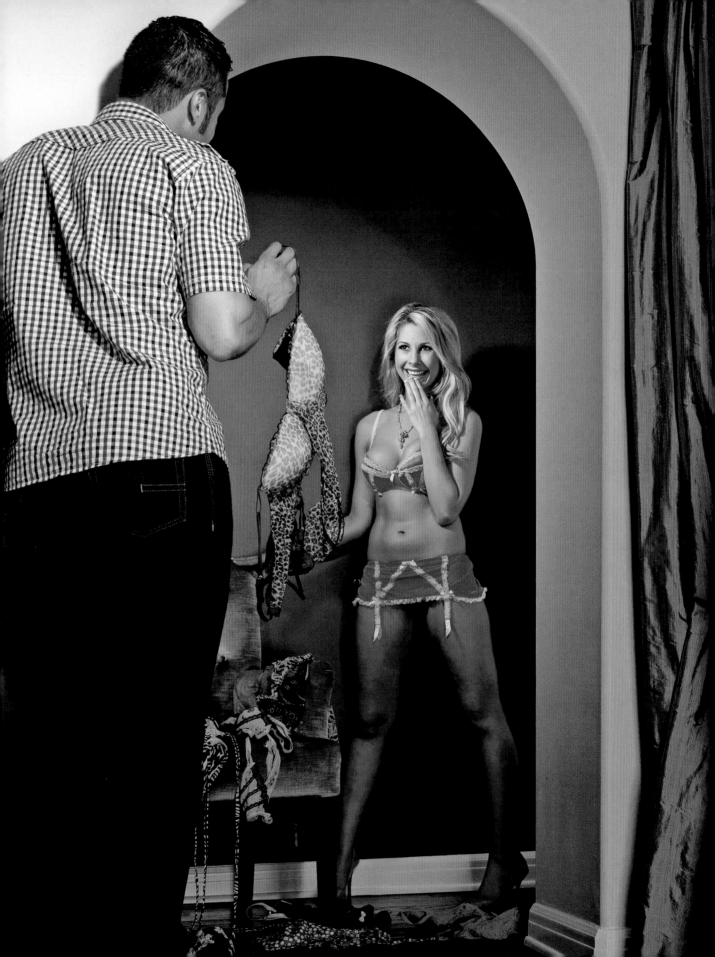

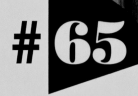

DRESSING ROOM ROMP

Guys get pretty annoyed when they have to wait outside the dressing room while you're trying on an outfit you probably won't buy anyway. To make shopping a lot less tedious for your man, invite him into the room ... where, of course, he'll find you ready for action.

....

Estimated time: 10 minutes
What you'll need: tissues, a dressing room with a security-locked door, a vow to keep your mounting excitement quiet

....

THE PLAY BY PLAY

1. Gals, get the room ready for your encounter before beckoning your guy to join you. Make sure all the store's merchandise is hung up and out of the way and there's no one close by.

2. "Darling," you call out in your sweetest voice. "Can you please come in and see if you like this? I'm just not sure about it." Before he's at your door, strip down to your bra and panties (lingerie preferred!).

3. As soon as he walks in the room, don't wait a nanosecond for his happy shock to register. Remind him to lock the door, then grab him by the belt, unzip his pants, kneel down, and yank out his prized possession.

4. Rather than go for the same old, same old blow job, switch it around. If you always use the sliding technique (where you slide your mouth up and down the penis), try varying it with some of these techniques ...

5. Use your tongue like a snake. Flicking your tongue back and forth over the head of his penis will really get him going because the head of the penis is the most sensitive area.

6. Speed up and then slow down. This will help produce more powerful orgasms and also prolong his ejaculation.

7. Since you're in the dressing room, for neatness's sake, it's probably a good idea to swallow. But if you're one of those ladies who just can't bear the taste, the trick is to do it without tasting. The most common response is to hold it in your mouth anticipating the swallow. What you need to do is swallow *immediately* and *hard*. This way the semen will go straight down without an aftertaste.

8. He'll happily wipe your mouth clean with grateful kisses.

9. Now send him on his way and make sure the dressing room is left in pristine condition. Use the tissues to wipe up any evidence.

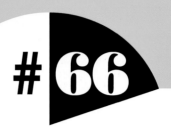

DOUBLE-DUTY FIREWORKS

There's nothing like brilliant fireworks accompanied by heart-pounding blasts and bangs to get you pumped to explode. Well, you're here, aren't you? Don't wait for the fuse to blow.

Estimated time: 5–7 minutes
What you'll need: a large blanket, lube

THE PLAY BY PLAY

1. The crowd is in a frenzy of excitement but you've both got your own reasons to be turned on.

2. While standing, wrap yourselves as snugly as two pigs in a blanket. Your lady should stand in front of you, facing away.

3. Hike her skirt with one hand and yank her panties down with the other. When she's exposed, unzip your pants and take out your works.

4. Pull the lube from your pocket and generously apply it to your cock and to her anus (if she's not comfortable with this, try a finger instead, or go the tried-and-true pussy route).

5. Rest your cock just on the edge of her anus (or vagina) but each time there's an explosion, insert yourself deeper and deeper inside her.

6. Have your lady time her reaction to the ooohs and aaahs of the crowd so that no one will notice her cries of ecstasy are anything other than a show of celebratory pleasure.

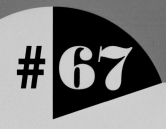

PHOTO-BOOTH BONER

Every now and then in shopping malls, you'll come across those little photo booths. *Hello?* Is there any better public place for fast and photogenic nookie? Bonus: You'll leave the booth with souvenir pictures chronicling your lust. Just be sure to pick a time when traffic is low— a lunch break rendezvous during the workday would be ideal.

Estimated time: 3–5 minutes. Be aware customers may be lining up outside.
What you'll need: a photo booth, lube, comfort in front of cameras

THE PLAY BY PLAY

1. As soon as you both enter, draw the curtain tightly closed and adjust the seats so that your laps can't be seen from outside the booth.

2. Then, ladies, lift your skirt and sit snugly on your man's exposed lap. If you're still dry, lube your pussy or ask your man to do the honors. Be assured no one walking by will have any clue about what's up.

3. Now move around on his lap and get him hard while you both keep one eye, if possible, on your reflections in the camera box.

4. Next, guide his penis through the back door into your vagina. Stay still and let him pick up his own rhythm and do the pumping. Meanwhile, keep your hands on the stool to keep it from shifting.

5. This might be a good time to slip your money in the slot and press "start." Expect the camera to start snapping away while your guy's excitement is mounting.

6. If you're easily stimulated, you may reach a climax with your lover. If not, consider it worth the adventure. And remember: Smile.

7. Don't forget to pick up your photos when you leave the booth!

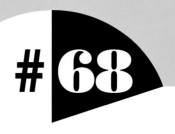

BEST BARGAIN IN TOWN

Time is money, and these days most of us are trying to save both. According to statistics, millions of people spend their weekend mornings searching for bargains at flea markets and yard sales. If you're one of them, change things up a bit and bring your erotic imagination along with those bags and wallet.

Estimated time: 3–5 minutes
What you'll need: a latex glove, a plastic bag, lube, an eagle eye, an out-of-the-way spot, a bondage prop

THE PLAY BY PLAY

1. Here's the game plan. Your first task is to hunt down something you can use for bondage play: rope, scarf, Halloween mask, wooden spoon, etc. Anything that looks gently used and fun to you will do the trick.

2. Once you've bought your prop, scope out the scene for a secluded spot away from other bargain hunters, such as down the street in a quiet park, or behind a deserted office building.

3. Gals, you're the dominatrix in this scenario. Depending on your prop, you can threaten, tickle, slap, or bind your "prey" into submission.

4. When your submissive guy is good and hot, pull out his penis and slip on the latex glove. Lube the glove slightly, but not too generously because you want to maintain some friction.

5. For a change of pace, open your palm and aggressively swirl it around the head, first in one direction then the other, before returning to a piston-pumping action. Keep the pressure firm and steady. You don't have all the time in the world to get him off—there's more deals to be had!

6. Be on the lookout for any stray shoppers. Yet at the same time be firm with your man. If he hesitates in any way or makes any sound, use your prop to keep him in line. Threats, accompanied by the sensation of the latex on his shaft, will arouse him quickly.

7. Once he's shot his wad, wrap your glove in a plastic bag and toss it in a nearby trashcan. But keep the prop in view to remind you both of your memorable booty bargain.

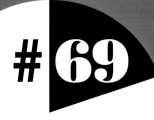

BUMP UP YOUR ETD

Instead of setting your watches to arrive precisely on schedule for an event—whether it's going to the theater for your Friday date night or going to pick up the kids from a sporting event—leave the house about 12 minutes early to play your own adult version of a car-ride game.

Estimated time: 5–7 minutes
What you'll need: your car, a relatively secluded area, lube

THE PLAY BY PLAY

1. Don't waste any time. While your guy is driving, remove your panties and place your legs on the dashboard. Start pleasuring your pussy by stroking your mound and labia and diddling your clit with your finger.

2. You don't want your driver to take his eyes off the road (safety comes first!) so describe with dirty talk what you're doing and how you're feeling. "Oh, my pussy is getting wet. I'm putting lots of greasy lube all over it. My lady wants your big hot rod inside her. Now!"

3. Then cry out, "Pull over before I come!"

4. Help him find a secluded area off the main road, turn off the headlights and park the car. Let him be the first to climb into the backseat. Scramble over the seat right after him.

5. Sit on top of his lap but face away from him so he can take in the scent of your hair and you can see out the windshield. Grab hold of the seats in front of you.

6. After he sticks his cock inside of your wet and juicy pussy, bounce up and down. It will only be a matter of minutes before you reach your destination.

7. Remember to check the car mirror to freshen your makeup. And guys, don't forget to zip up!

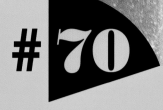

#70

LOCKER ROOM ANTICS

Be daring and hit the showers together after working up a nice sweat at the gym. You're better off in the guy's locker room because they're less likely to scream out if they catch you—heck, they might even be into it.

Estimated time: 10 minutes
What you'll need: a deserted locker room, a baseball cap, a private shower stall, two generously sized towels or robes kept within reach, a change of clothes

THE PLAY BY PLAY

1. Choose a low-traffic gym time. If it's a 24-hour establishment, late in the night or very early in the AM is probably best. Ladies, you may want to keep a baseball cap on your head to be a little more incognito for later on.

2. Work out together side-by-side to build up the heat. Guys, flex your pecs flirtatiously. Ladies, strut your stuff by doing those thigh crunches while looking seductively at your man. Spot each other if necessary.

3. After a strenuous workout, it's time to wash off your sweat. Why separate now? Guys, scope out your locker room first to be sure it's not crowded. Leave your towels and clothes in a shower stall.

4. All clear? Ladies, pull your hat down and sneak in with your man. Once you're in, get those dirty clothes off!

5. The shower offers the perfect opportunity to engage in the "bent overs." Turn your lovely around and get her to rest her hands on the tiles or hold onto the soap rack. Make sure she feels supported before you enter her. If you have any doubts, ask her in a whisper if she feels safe.

6. After your release, offer her oral sex while you're still in the shower. Women especially love it when you go down on them here because they're comfortable knowing their vagina is as clean as a whistle—and having a hot tongue salivating on their clit while an intense stream of water is pouring down only amplifies the pleasure.

7. After she's climaxed, soap up and rinse one another off with playful abandon. In case anyone is nearby, be sure to stifle your squeals of delight.

8. Now shut the water off, grab those towels and dry each other while you're still in the stall. Dress one another there too. Careful not to slip!

9. Even if a fellow gym goer catches a glance of your woman as you're heading out, it's no biggie. Just say she walked in to grab her towel—it won't be a lie!

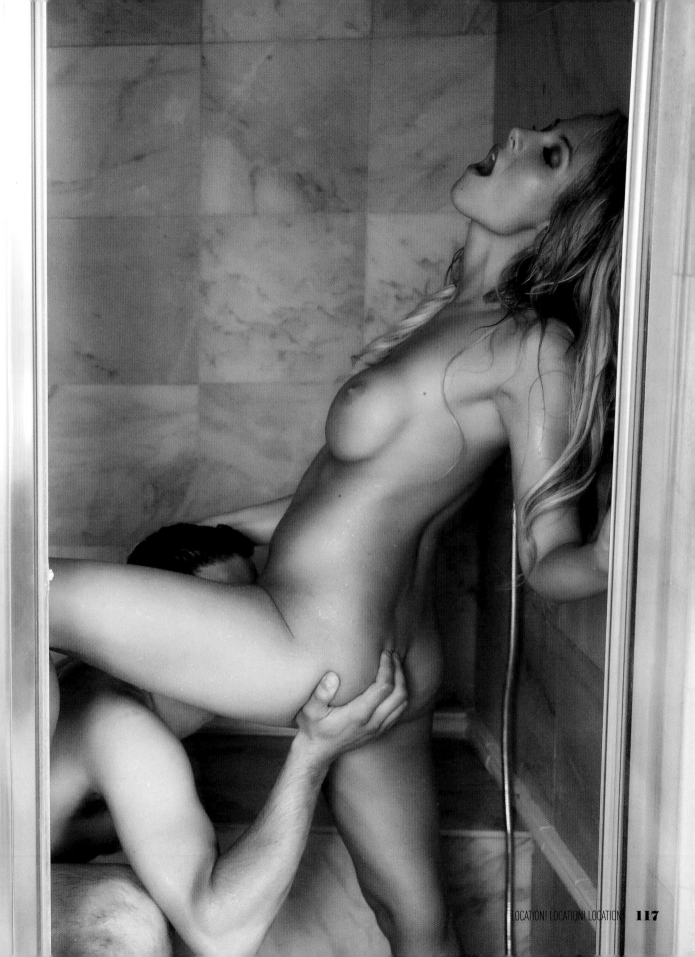

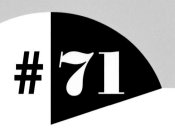

SHOPPING FOR FURNITURE

Thinking of feathering your nest? Get rid of pesky salespeople by telling them you're just looking, then try out the goods—from bedding and sofas to a reclining chair.

Estimated time: 10–12 minutes
What you'll need: one eye on your surroundings, a furniture store with salespeople who leave you alone, willingness to expose your wild side

THE PLAY BY PLAY

1. If you've got a touch of the exhibitionist, you'll definitely get a kick out of having sex on display furniture.

2. Plan your erotic adventure in advance, and wear no undergarments. Women, choose a skirt; men, lose jeans.

3. Scope out the store and single out those pieces of furniture that are the most inviting. But don't linger for too long on any one item because a salesperson might zoom in.

4. Turn the heat up by first lying on a bed and staring into each other's eyes—no touching.

5. Then move to a sofa. Sit next to each other and rub your lover's genitals. When you can't stand it anymore, move to a reclining chair. If it has a built-in massager, so much the better.

6. Girlfriends, now is not the time to be shy. Sit on his lap and pull out his cock. Slip it into your wet pussy.

7. Move with care and quiet. Squirm ever so slightly. Perhaps he can fiddle with the reclining mechanism, bringing the chair up and down and back and forth until his erection is bursting, at the same time feeling the vibrations of the auto-matic massager, if the chair has one.

8. Even though the sensations are thrilling, chances are, under these conditions, you won't have an orgasm. But don't despair; reliving your sexual exploits later in the day will have you primed for fantastic oral or manual sex once you're home.

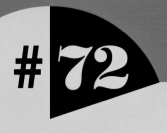

SENSATIONAL SPRINKLER

It's pitch dark and the only sounds are crickets and the whirl of the automatic sprinkler—now it's time to add your moans. Make the most out of the time it takes to water your backyard lawn: Instead of using a hose (although that could be fun, too!), opt for a sprinkler so you can multitask. Make sure the kids are fast asleep too!

Estimated time: 8–10 minutes
What you'll need: a hot day; a sprinkler with a steady, whirling spray; a secluded area

THE PLAY BY PLAY

1. When the summer temperature is sky-high and the thought of relief from the cool spray of a sprinkler is an irresistible idea, grab your partner and strip down until you're both completely bare.

2. Run and frolic through the spray as if you are two carefree children. Play releases feel-good endorphins that set the stage for superexciting sex.

3. When all tension is released, ladies, take the plunge and bend over so the water hits your genitals. If you can't reach your hands to the ground, just place them on your thighs or calves for support so you can remain steady and open to the sensations.

4. Guys, once you see that your lady is almost near orgasm as she gyrates to the sputtering water against her clit, stand behind her and put your hands around her waist. Keep the water pointed toward her, but not you.

5. By now she should be wet and receptive and wholly open to a rear-entry pump. Go for it. The double stimulation (for her) should maximize the opportunity to climax in unison.

6. This supersensual experience is also heightened by the aroma of wet grass, the feel of hot air against skin, the pulsation of the cool water, and the sounds of the whooshing sprinkler. Don't be surprised if you both yearn to repeat the experience on the next sultry day.

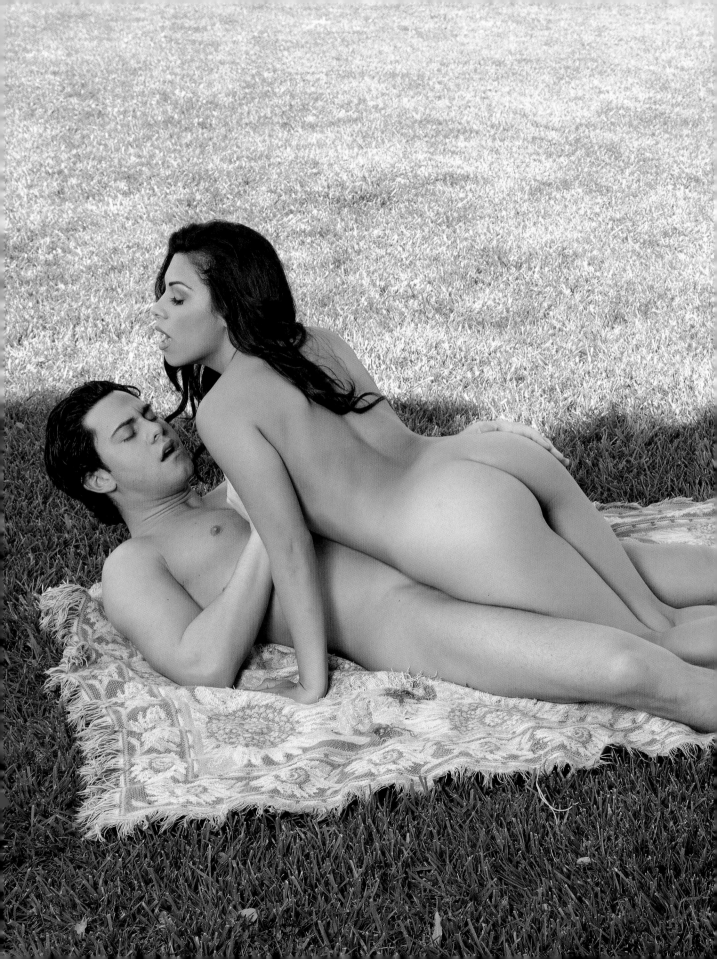

HOLE IN ONE

For those busy couples who like to swing their clubs, here's what's so great about having sex on the golf course: (1) You've already booked the time, (2) The grass is soft, and there are no rocks or twigs on the ground, and (3) It could improve your "game."

Estimated time: 5 minutes or less
What you'll need: a secluded area, time when the course isn't packed, lube, some golf clubs, a jacket or blanket

THE PLAY BY PLAY

1. As soon as you find yourselves alone on the course (or far away from anyone's view), take advantage of the opportunity and throw down your jackets or blanket on a smooth, grassy patch.

2. It's always a good idea to keep it simple because you never know when another golfer is going to appear, so opt for the woman-on-top position, which promises the fastest orgasms.

3. Ladies, if you're in a hurry, lie down with your legs between your man's and keep them very close together. His penis will be squeezed in a way that makes it hard to move into any other sexual position. Even though he is likely to ejaculate quickly in this position, it creates unrivaled feelings of intimacy and connection. For a woman who likes the sense of penetration and the feeling of her man's penis inside her, this is a powerful hole-in-one experience.

4. Variations on the woman-on-top positions are all about the angle of the penis in the vagina, and the fact that you get different sensations when your guy penetrates you from different angles. This can be exciting for your man as well, of course, because different positions stimulate different parts of his penis and also put different degrees of pressure on it.

5. In any case, be as quick about it as possible because the likelihood of a golf ball sailing your way is on par with the pleasure of the experience.

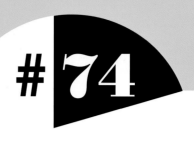

GET TO WORK

Employ this superhot scenario to give his workday a whole new meaning. Just be absolutely sure the coast is clear, the door can be locked, and there will be no interruptions. Try a Friday night after all of the staff has left, and tell your man you'll come pick him up.

Estimated time: 5 minutes
What you'll need: a blindfold, a scarf, pantyhose, a brown-bag lunch or folder with papers

THE PLAY BY PLAY

1. As soon as you enter the office, lock the door and tell him to stay seated. Then walk behind his chair and blindfold him.

2. Climb out of your clothes and use them to tie him to his seat. Panties, bra, scarves, and pantyhose can work as binders.

3. Next, straddle him and move back and forth across his lap like you've got an itch that needs to be scratched. Why stop there? Slip your erect nipples into his mouth. If he protests, be firm and say in a commanding whisper, "Be quiet or I won't set you free."

4. Now slide down to the floor and get on your knees. Kiss his inner thighs and then head up to his cock.

5. Hold the base and, in the lightest, gentlest way, take the head into your mouth. Keeping the tip of your tongue soft, tenderly lick the tip.

6. As soon as he's hard and ready to burst, cup your hand over his mouth. Even if he bites your palm, continue to apply pressure, sending the message that it's not okay to make any noise. Now continue sucking until your job is done.

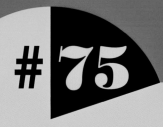

BEACH BALLING

If you've managed to find time for a few hours at the beach, you've hit the erotic jackpot. The beach is a natural seductress. The sun triggers our feel-good endorphin levels and the ocean's roar awakens our senses.

Estimated time: 12 minutes (the beach atmosphere slows down biorhythms)
What you'll need: a blanket or a couple huge beach towels; an umbrella (optional), cooler with cans of soft drinks, sunscreen

THE PLAY BY PLAY

1. Lay down on your blankets carefully, allowing them to cover as much ground area as possible. Hot sand on sensative skin can be uncomfortable, and you want to avoid getting it in an irritating place like the vagina. The friction could lead to a broken condom if you're using one.

2. Strategically place the cooler so it's within reach while also shielding you from public view.

3. Take turns spreading sunscreen on each other, continuing to rub it all over your lover's body.

4. Guys, while your bathing beauty is lolling in the warmth of the sun, give her a thrill. Open the cooler and grab an icy can. Now surprise her by rubbing it along her back and inside her thighs. Then roll it around on her mound, over her bathing suit bottom. Expect squeals of protest.

5. So much for just laying back and enjoying lazy, languid lovemaking. You've charged up your lady.

6. Now is the time. There's no need to strip down. Just pull your bathing suits to the side and diddle each other. Keep this up for as long as you like until you feel the unstoppable urge to go all the way. But be discreet. If you have an umbrella tip it in such a way that privacy is ensured. Or wrap the blanket around you so you're completely covered.

7. You can also do it in the water if you'd rather (or in addition) if the beach is deserted. Guys, all you have to do is sit at the edge of the water (no deeper), knees up, with your lover sitting facing you, her legs wrapped around your waist. As the tide goes in and out, so do you. Get swept away in the magic of it all.

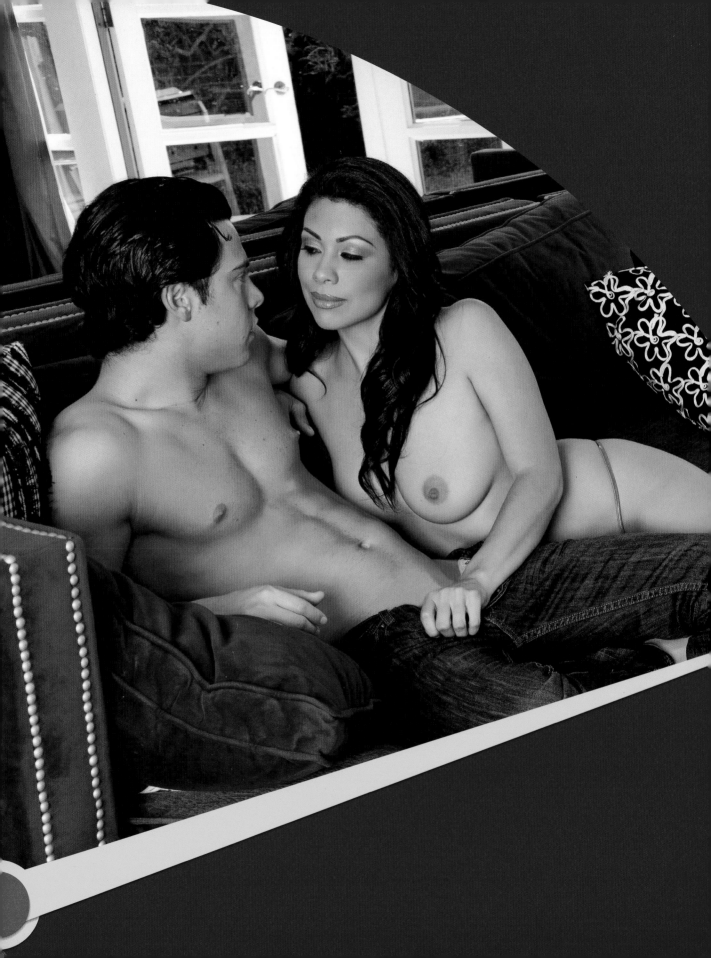

ACKNOWLEDGMENTS

Tremendous gratitude to the creative and hardworking team at Quiver Books, especially Will Kiester, Amanda Waddell, Meg Sniegoski, Holly Randall, and Traffic Design Consultants, for publishing this exquisite and informative resource.

I'd also like to offer boundless appreciation to my dozens of friends and family members, writing buddies, yogis, hair salon confidantes, meditators, fellow supermarket shoppers, neighbors, gym-goers, and chatty eavesdropping strangers on the street, who candidly offered their diverse personal experiences and suggestions. All assured me there are endless ways time-crunched couples can have great sex and make their relationships even better.

Also a big hug to my husband, Dr. Bebop, a gifted cornet player who knows how to jazz up our love life with perfect rhythm, swinging riffs, imagination, tender embraces, a bottomless well of compassion, and all the time in the world: *Howie, without your support, where would I be?*

And finally, thank you to all those loving couples who believe in the enduring power of sexual connection and keep it a priority in their on-the-go lives.

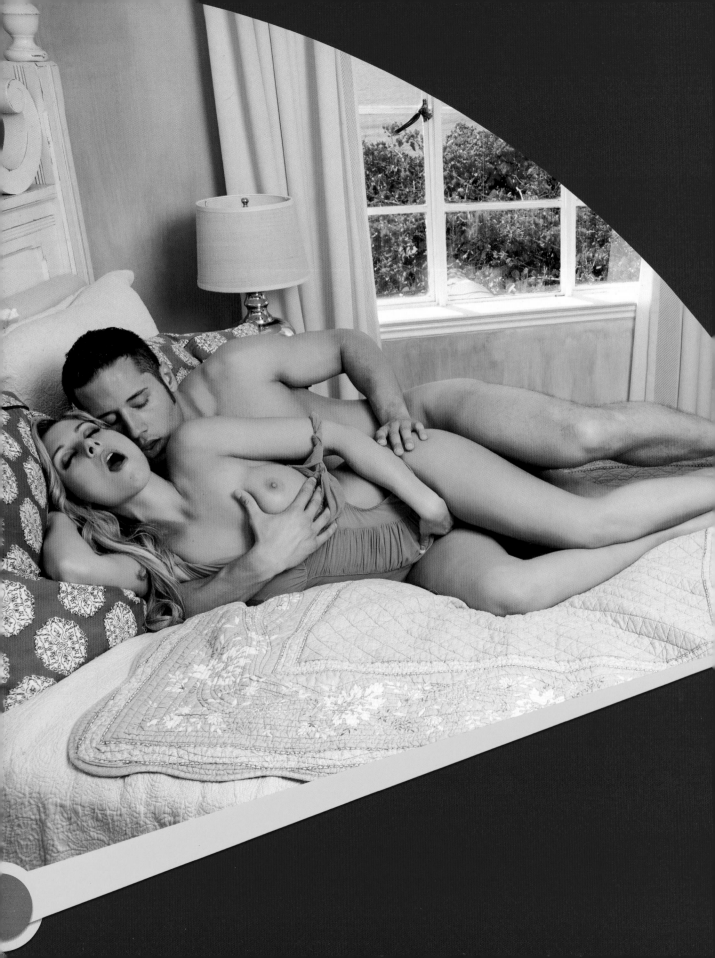

ABOUT THE AUTHOR

Robin Westen is an expert sex-advice columnist and journalist, with more than twenty years of experience writing for magazines such as *Glamour*, *Cosmopolitan*, *Family Circle*, *Ladies' Home Journal*, *Self*, *Good Housekeeping*, and more. She specializes in health, relationships, sex issues, and parenting.

Westen has authored several books and was an Emmy Award–winning writer for ABC's women's health–oriented show *FYI* and for *One Life to Live*. She is also a sex-advice columnist (Sex Rx) for *Woman's Own* magazine. Westen lives in Brooklyn and spends her summers in Vermont with her husband and son.